**DO NOT REMOVE
CARDS FROM POCKET**

Your Personalized Health Profile

Your Personalized Health Profile

CHOOSING THE DIET THAT'S RIGHT FOR YOU

Myron Winick, M.D.

William Morrow and Company, Inc.
New York

Library of Congress Cataloging in Publication Data

Winick, Myron.
 Your personalized health profile.

 Includes index.
 1. Diet therapy. 2. Nutrition. 3. Health.
I. Title. [DNLM: 1. Diet—popular works. 2. Food
Habits—popular works. 3. Health. 4. Nutrition—
popular works. 5. Probability—popular works.
QU 145 W772y]
RM216.W74 1985   613.2   85-7293
ISBN 0-688-05114-6

Printed in the United States of America

First Edition

1 2 3 4 5 6 7 8 9 10

BOOK DESIGN BY PATTY LOWY

Contents

2268459

Introduction

Myron Winick, M.D.

From many different sources we have been hearing that the American diet is not as balanced as it should be. Most experts now believe that our diet is too high in calories, too high in total fat and saturated fat, and too high in sodium and refined sugar. At the same time, our diet is too low in polyunsaturated fat, too low in starch, too low in fiber, and often too low in certain vitamins and minerals. These conclusions have led to a series of recommendations designed to improve our diet. These recommendations include:

- Reducing calories
- Reducing total fat from 40 percent to 30 percent of calories
- Reducing saturated fat to no more than one-half the total fat
- Reducing sodium to 5 grams or less
- Reducing refined sugar to 10 percent or less of total calories
- Increasing polyunsaturated fat to one-half the total fat
- Increasing complex carbohydrate (starch) to 50 percent or more of calories
- Increasing dietary fiber to 10 grams per day

7

- Increasing foods rich in such minerals as calcium, iron, and zinc, and such vitamins as vitamin A and folic acid

These recommendations would surely not harm anyone and would almost certainly reduce the incidence of some of our major diseases. Thus, the recommendations, which are based on the best scientific evidence presently available, are worthy of serious consideration by all of us. Unfortunately, we are all creatures of habit. And no habits are more ingrained and more difficult to change than eating habits. The way we eat is determined by our families, our ethnic backgrounds, our life-styles, and perhaps more than anything, our taste preferences. It's impractical to believe that overnight, Americans will give up hamburgers, or that Japanese and Chinese will stop using soy sauce. The incentive to change one's diet has to be great enough to make the self-discipline involved worth imposing. This book is designed to provide that incentive to at least a large number of people. By deciding quantitatively whether you are at high, moderate, or low risk for any of the serious nutritionally related diseases discussed in the following chapters, you can decide whether dietary modification is important for you.

Remember at the outset, however, that I am not advocating complacency or a false sense of security to those at low risk. Even those at lowest risk for a given disease may end up suffering from that disease. Your chances are just less than those of someone at higher risk. What I am saying is that if your risk is high, your incentive for modifying your diet should be as great. The diseases I will be discussing are all serious diseases. Modifying your diet may well reduce your chances of getting one or more of them. It is definitely something to think about seriously.

I am not saying that those of you who consume the "typical" American diet don't need to institute changes if your risk is low. I certainly hope that you would do so, because from a health standpoint you have nothing to lose and you might gain a great deal. I am saying also that those of you who are at high risk have even more to gain. Even if you modify your diet, there are no guarantees that you won't contract one of these diseases. What I can promise is that you will be less likely to get one than if you continued on the typical American diet. How much less likely would this be? I wish I could tell you exactly, but I can't. What I can tell you, however, is that the higher your risk, the greater your potential benefit.

Beyond your own health there is a second reason to modify your typical American diet: the effect it can have on those around you. When one person in a family must change his or her diet for health reasons, the importance of diet to maintaining proper health becomes evident to the other family members. Even more important, there is a direct "spin-off." The family begins to change its overall eating pattern and slowly all the members begin to eat in a manner that is closer to the recommended diet pattern. Soon it becomes obvious that these changes are neither difficult nor unpleasant. In fact, often new experiences are discovered which are more enjoyable than the old. A person who has reduced his salt intake often cannot enjoy salty food anymore. People who used to sweeten coffee and tea not only learn to add less sugar or even to eliminate it completely, but also to enjoy doing without. This change in eating pattern even among those who are not at high risk, and particularly the young, is extremely important because it is they who will set future trends and it is they who will soon be starting their own families and determining their children's eating patterns.

There are enough people at high risk for one or more of the diseases discussed in this book to wield collective power. The food industry is the largest single industry in the United States and it is very consumer-oriented. As more and more people begin to modify their diets, more and more food products will become available reflecting this changing pattern. The widespread use of vegetable oils and margarine is due in part to public concern over too much saturated fat in the diet. Concern about too much salt has been leading to many more products processed without salt. The more of these products that are available, the easier it is to modify your diet. Today even the best restaurants serve items compatible with the dietary recommendations made in this book. People at high risk for such serious diseases as atherosclerosis, high blood pressure, obesity, diabetes, certain cancers, osteoporosis, and some nutrient deficiencies can modify their diets without radically altering their life-styles. The more of you who try it the easier it will become.

Each chapter of this book is devoted to a serious illness that has as one of its major risk factors an improper diet. None of the diseases discussed is caused *solely* by poor diet. However, to the extent that diet is involved, you can modify it, often by taking rather simple steps, and lower your risk. As we shall see, many of the risk factors for these diseases are beyond our control. There is nothing any of us can do to change them. However, a few are under our control, and diet is one. If you are at high risk, you stand to gain directly if your diet needs to be changed. Do it soon; the longer you wait, the greater your risk!

Chapter 1

Your Nutrition Profile

The concept of being at risk for one or more diseases is not a new one. Insurance companies base their rates in part on assessed risk. Women pay lower premiums for life insurance than men because women live longer. Drivers under twenty-five pay more for automobile insurance because they are involved in more accidents than older drivers. Thus, if you are in a high-risk group you pay a higher premium even if you are a very careful driver.

When it comes to *preventing* specific diseases, deciding who is at risk is much more difficult. First, the population at risk must be defined. Second, members of that population must be identified. Third, reasonable preventive measures must be available. Fourth, the population at risk must be induced to take these preventive measures.

Let us follow a specific disease to see how one or more problems might develop in applying this concept. AIDS (acquired immune deficiency syndrome) is a disease that is currently frightening most of us. It destroys the immune system, and one-third of those it strikes die. At present, the populations at risk seem fairly well defined—homosexuals, drug users, and people who require repeated blood transfusions. What is not clear, and therefore is cause for wide concern, is whether the risk of this infectious disease will remain confined to these populations. Hence,

11

defining the population at risk is not as simple as it may seem, and particularly if the disease is infectious, that population may be constantly changing. Even if we limit ourselves to the populations cited, some members of certain of these groups may not wish it known that they are members, particularly if such an admission is viewed as self-incriminating. Thus, actually reaching all the people at risk may be extremely difficult. Assuming they could all be reached, we do not know the cause of AIDS, and there is no specific preventive measure presently available, no vaccine, no serum, no medicine that will render an individual immune. But let us hope that very soon a vaccine will be available. How safe will it be? Even the most innocuous vaccines can cause illness and even death. Finally, how do all those at risk get vaccinated? Does society request it or does society demand it?

As complicated as this sequence may appear, it has been very effective in preventing many of the most devastating infectious diseases. Smallpox, polio, diphtheria, measles, whooping cough, and tetanus have been all but eliminated in the United States. Influenza, while still fairly common, is much better controlled because people at risk for serious complications (the elderly and those with a chronic illness) can be identified, reached, and vaccinated. In fact, the preventive approach has had its greatest success with those diseases which are caused by a specific infectious agent, and for which a safe and effective vaccine is available. Since these diseases are infectious, literally all people at risk must be immunized; therefore, many who would not themselves have gotten the infections must submit to preventive measures. In this situation the individual undergoes some discomfort, and even takes a small risk, for the good of society.

The principles of preventive medicine are just now beginning to be applied to nutrition to protect populations at risk. Many diseases are caused in part by a lifelong pattern of eating—too many calories, too much fat, too much salt, too little complex carbohydrate, or too little dietary fiber. However, in many ways it is even more difficult to use the principles outlined above to prevent nutritional disease than to prevent an infectious disease.

Defining the Population at Risk

A number of the most serious diseases in our society are at least partly due to long-term dietary patterns. Atherosclerosis, high blood pressure, obesity, cancer, diabetes, chronic vitamin and mineral deficiencies, certain diseases of the gastrointestinal tract, and abnormalities of bones and teeth all fall into this category. Are you at risk for one or more of these diseases? And if so, how high is that risk? These two questions must be answered as fully as possible before you can make a really informed decision whether or not a change in diet is necessary. In a few instances the answers may be simple. For example, if you are a man, the chance of developing breast cancer is extremely low—much too low to consider any major dietary change. In most instances, however, the answers are much less clear. They depend on your sex, your race, your ancestry, your life-style, and your environment, and on the diet you have been consuming most of your life. Let us take high blood pressure (hypertension). If you are black, your risk is higher than if you are white; if you are male, your risk is slightly higher than if you are female; if you have a strong family history, your risk is increased; if your life-style produces constant pressure, your risk goes up; and if you eat foods that are relatively high in salt, you are more likely to have high blood pressure.

It should be clear that establishing a *precise* risk for any individual is nearly impossible. While you know without question whether you are male or female, black or white, it is much more difficult to know whether you have a strong family history, a pressured life-style, or whether you consume a high-salt diet. What constitutes a strong family history? Certainly high blood pressure in one distant cousin on your maternal grandmother's side does not. And just as certainly, if your mother and father, both sets of grandparents, and all your siblings have high blood pressure, this does. But what about the middle ground? One grandparent and an uncle? Both grandparents on your mother's side? One grandparent on each side? And what is a pressured life-style? Policeman, executive, coal miner, firefighter? Going through a divorce? Suffering the loss of a loved one? Finally, do you eat a high-salt diet? How high is high? Americans eat a lot of salt, but the Japanese eat more. Salt is ubiquitous; it is introduced into our food supply through all kinds of processing. Canned peas may contain one hundred times as much salt as fresh peas. Sodium, the active ingredient in salt, is added not only to many processed foods, but also to many over-the-counter medicines. Thus, most of us do not have any idea how much sodium we consume, let alone whether we are consuming *too much*.

For that reason, establishing your exact (absolute) risk is usually impossible. However, it is easier to establish your relative risk (how high yours is compared with the average person's), and classifying yourself at high risk, moderate risk, or low risk is often possible. To do this, however, you must take into account your sex and your race, and you must carefully assess your family background, your lifestyle, your environment, and your diet. Only then can you answer the question, am I at high risk for any of the diet-related diseases?

Your Sex

After the adolescent years, nutrient deficiencies occur almost solely in women, rarely in men. Some studies suggest that as many as one-half of all American women are depleted to some extent in at least one of the vitamins or minerals. Why do women find themselves in this predicament and what can they do to avoid it? During the reproductive years, women cycle between pregnancy, lactation, and the long periods in between. Pregnancy and lactation impose increased demands for certain nutrients. Unless special care is taken, deficiencies can and will occur. During the interim periods, women lose a significant amount of blood each month. Blood loss means iron loss. It also means that new red cells must be made, and this process requires larger amounts of certain nutrients.

Two characteristics of the life-styles of women in our society also increase their risk for certain deficiencies. Women are often dieting, limiting their calories, and in so doing, they are also limiting their intake of certain essential nutrients. And many women are regular users of oral contraceptives, which may interfere with the absorption and metabolism of certain vitamins. In addition, women are rapidly approaching men in their consumption of alcohol, another agent known to reduce the absorption of several vitamins and minerals. Thus, the modern American woman who is taking oral contraceptives, consuming moderate amounts of alcohol, constantly watching her weight, and often crash dieting is at particular risk for nutrient deficiencies.

Finally, women undergo certain hormonal changes later in life that constitute the menopause. Along with the well-known manifestations of menopause are less well-known changes in a woman's body chemistry. These changes increase her needs for at least one nutrient, calcium.

If you are a woman, you are automatically at greater risk for nutrient deficiencies than if you are a man. In addition, cancer of the breast and of the uterus, two very serious diseases, are related to long-term dietary patterns.

From the discussion so far, it might seem that women are more at risk than men are for nutritionally related disease. In fact, this is not true. If anything, it is the reverse. Men die more often from heart attacks than women do, and heart attack is the number one killer in America today. Thus, although atherosclerosis occurs in both sexes, it is more common in men. Since both obesity and diabetes can lead to atherosclerosis, these two diseases, although no more frequent in men than in women, are more serious in men.

Therefore, *which* sex is more at risk is not the question. For certain problems women are; for others, men are. What *is* important is that when you assess your own personal risk, you factor your sex into the equation.

Your Race

Simply belonging to a particular racial group can increase your risk for certain diseases. Blacks are more prone to sickle-cell anemia than whites or Orientals are. By contrast, thalassemia, another deadly form of anemia, is more common in whites, particularly those of Mediterranean background. Cystic fibrosis, a very serious disease involving the gastrointestinal tract and the lungs, is seen almost exclusively in Caucasians of Eastern European background. These diseases are genetically induced, and as far as we know, are unrelated to diet. Certain diseases, however, which are clearly related to nutrition are also more common in one race than in another. In this case the person's genetic makeup renders him more susceptible to the effects of the offending diet.

The two most important conditions in which your genetic makeup may play a part are hypertension (high blood pressure), which is much more prevalent in blacks than in whites, and lactose intolerance (inability to digest milk sugar), which is extremely severe in Orientals, moderately so in blacks, and much less so in Caucasians. Thus, if you are black and living in the United States, your risk for hypertension is increased and you must be particularly careful to minimize the other risk factors for this disease. If you are Oriental or black, your risk for *lactose intolerance* is high and you may have to control the amount of milk and dairy products in your diet.

We are not certain why these two conditions show racial preferences, and in the case of high blood pressure, we are not even certain that its increased incidence in blacks is entirely due to genetic factors. However, it is quite clear that blacks and Orientals must take race into account when determining their risk for these two important nutritionally related conditions.

Your Family History

Many of us know the small town where our great-grandparents were born even if it was in a distant country. Some of us even know our great-grandfather's occupation. But how many know how old he was when he died and from what cause? As for our grandparents, probably few of us could say with any certainty whether Grandmother had high blood pressure and even fewer, how high it was.

Even those who are able to trace their family back many generations, and who can reveal such details about distant relatives as their occupation, education, and religion, know very little about these relatives' health and almost nothing about their specific health problems. People almost consciously avoid asking about illnesses and even when told, tend to put such information out of their minds. Yet this knowledge could be crucial in helping them predict their own risk for heart attack, high blood pressure, diabetes, and many other diseases.

The crucial nutritionally related diseases in which family history is important are: *atherosclerosis,* which may lead to heart attack or coronary artery disease, kidney disease, and senility; *high blood pressure* (hypertension), which can cause stroke or cerebral vascular accidents (CVA), heart failure, and kidney disease; *diabetes,* which may lead to atherosclerosis and all its complications as well as to kidney failure, decreased feeling in fingers and toes (peripheral neuropathy), blindness, and weakness of the extremities; *obesity,* which is associated with atherosclerosis, hypertension, and diabetes as well as with gall bladder disease; certain bone diseases such as *osteoporosis,* which can cause fractures of the hip and vertebrae in later life.

While we will discuss several other important diseases that are related to diet and for which your risk may be lowered by instituting certain dietary modifications, those mentioned above are the most important to trace when taking your family history. Sometimes just asking what Grandfather died from will supply the answer; more often, you may have to dig. Relatives may not remember the disease but may remember certain consequences of it. The more information you can gather, the better you can build your family "health tree."

For close living relatives, the direct approach is often the most productive. Do they have *atherosclerosis*? Have they ever had a *heart attack* or heart pains *(angina)*? What is their blood pressure? If they don't know, were they ever told it was high? If they have never had their blood pressure taken, suggest that they do so. Did they ever have a *stroke,* even a mild one? Were they ever told they had *heart failure*? Were they short of breath when climbing two flights of stairs or less? Was it more difficult to breathe when lying flat than when propped up with two pillows? Do they currently take heart pills—nitroglycerine or digitalis? Do they take diuretics? Have they been told to limit their salt intake? Do they have diabetes? High blood sugar? Sugar in the urine? Do they take *insulin* or *oral hypoglycemic drugs*? Are they extremely overweight? Were they overweight in the past? Did the female members of the family become shorter in old age? Did any of them fracture a hip or a wrist? Were they ever told they had osteoporosis? These are the important questions to ask. Be persistent. Get the answers! From the answers a family pattern may emerge that will help you determine whether you are at increased risk for one or more diet-related diseases.

Below is a checklist containing the most important family health information you must have when you try to trace your family health tree to see whether it shows those diseases that have a major nutritional component in their cause.

- Atherosclerosis: heart attack, angina, blood pressure, stroke, heart failure, shortness of breath, nitroglycerine, digitalis, diuretics, told to limit salt
- Diabetes: insulin, special "diabetic" diet, numbness or loss of power in extremities, kidney disease, blindness
- Obesity: actual weight of relatives
- Osteoporosis: shorter during old age; fractured hip or wrist
- Hypertension: high blood pressure, rise in blood pressure with age, heart attack, stroke, kidney disease

If you are seeking information about a relative who has died, you may have to use several sources, particularly if the death occurred some time ago. Ask your grandparents about their parents. If your grandparents are dead, can one of their brothers or sisters supply the information you need? Discuss the health of your grandparents with your own parents and with your uncles and aunts. The most important relatives are those listed in the health tree.

Once you have gathered all the information available, you must put it together to see if a pattern emerges. Let us examine the "big four" family-related nutritional diseases: atherosclerosis, hypertension, diabetes, and obesity. First, separate those you definitely know have one or more of these diseases from those who are presumed, from complications or symptoms, to have or have had them. Thus, your mother's mother may have been definitely obese and may be presumed to have had hypertension because she had a stroke and died of heart failure. Your mother's father may have definitely had high blood pressure; he died of a heart attack after suffering from angina for many years and so is presumed to have had atherosclerosis. Your father's father died of a heart attack (he is presumed to have had atherosclerosis). Your father's mother died in an

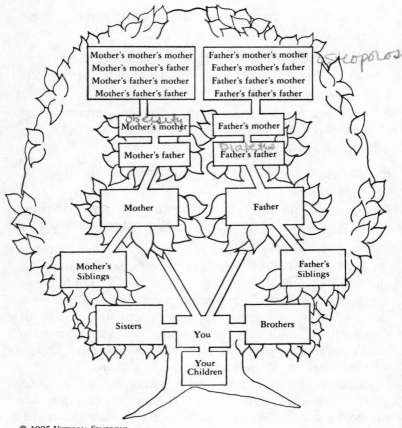

Mother's mother's mother
Mother's mother's father
Mother's father's mother
Mother's father's father

Father's mother's mother
Father's mother's father
Father's father's mother
Father's father's father

Mother's mother

Father's mother

Mother's father

Father's father

Mother

Father

Mother's Siblings

Father's Siblings

Sisters

Brothers

You

Your Children

accident. Your mother was obese, had hypertension, and died of a stroke. Your father died of a brain tumor, but had had a mild coronary several years before. One of your three siblings is obese.

Your tree is shown on page 21.

Clearly, both high blood pressure and obesity are common on your mother's side of the family. Atherosclerosis is presumed to have occurred on both sides of the family, and diabetes is absent. The closer the disease is to you on the tree, the more important a risk factor it is for you. Thus,

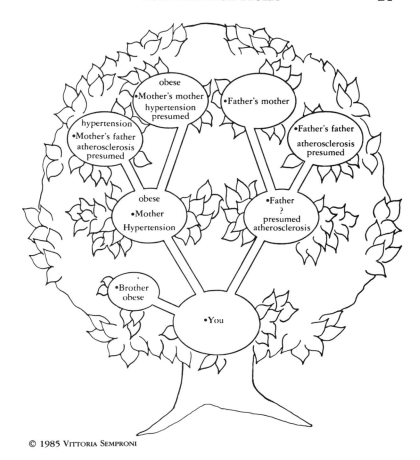

© 1985 Vittoria Semproni

obesity and hypertension are definite risk factors even though they do not appear on your father's side. You have already learned a lot. As we shall see in Chapter 3, you are already at high enough risk for high blood pressure to lower your salt intake, and if you are black, that risk is even higher. Your risk for obesity is also high enough for you to watch your calories, particularly because you are prone to hypertension and obesity can lead to hypertension. As for atherosclerosis, you just cannot be sure. Examining your family tree further may uncover more information. If it does not, the issue remains in doubt.

If all your other risk factors are negative, dietary modification aimed at preventing atherosclerosis is probably not necessary. If, however, you have other risk factors, your suspicious family history will tip the scales even more. The history I have outlined above, or some variation of it, is not unusual. In fact, it is close to my own family history. And I watch my weight and calories and consume a moderately salt-restricted diet. Your own history may present a much different pattern, perhaps better, perhaps worse, but whatever pattern emerges, it is important to know about it. For once your health tree is carefully constructed, you have taken the first step in determining your risk for four of the most serious diseases in our society. This risk, if it is high, can be altered by a particular dietary pattern.

Life-style
Perhaps even more important than your sex, race, or family history in determining whether you are at risk for certain nutritionally related diseases, is your life-style. People who live under constant pressure, whether real or imaginary (so-called Type A personalities), are at increased risk for atherosclerosis and hypertension. Smoking increases your risk for atherosclerosis. Drinking and using a variety of drugs will also increase your risk for certain nutrient deficiencies, particularly if you are a woman. Constant dieting will not only limit calories, but may limit the intake of important nutrients and, when carried to extremes, may result in overt deficiencies. By contrast, moderate amounts of exercise not only will increase the efficiency of your heart and lungs, but may also lower your risk for atherosclerosis and its complications. It is extremely important in assessing your risk for certain important nutritionally related diseases that you examine your life-style honestly. If it is increasing your risk perhaps it can be altered. Even if this is not possible, knowing the increased risk will al-

low you to make an informed decision as to whether a change in your diet may be helpful.

Type A Personality

More than twenty years ago an association was made between a particular set of behavioral characteristics and coronary artery disease. People who exhibited this set of characteristics were labeled as having Type A personalities. They were described as being intensely ambitious, extremely competitive, constantly preoccupied with occupational deadlines, and often consumed by a sense of urgency. Type A behavior is a state of mental arousal characterized by a competitive, ambitious, hard-driving existence. Don't confuse this behavior pattern with simply working hard or with achieving success. It resembles more a constant striving toward accomplishment. Thus, Type A behavior involves a series of personality traits coupled with an environment that transforms those traits into a stressful existence. Such behavior is associated with an increased incidence of atherosclerosis and hypertension, and is a major risk factor in these two diseases.

Do you have a Type A personality? It may not be easy to answer that question objectively since it is often difficult to perceive one's own personality. There are questionnaires that can be used, but to decide whether your behavior pattern constitutes a major, moderate or low-risk pattern, an objective assessment by your spouse or a close friend is often enough. Does your wife perceive you as constantly driven, always under pressure from your job or outside influences? Does your husband see you as always under pressure from self-imposed deadlines that create a sense of urgency even if it does not really exist? If the answer is a definite yes, you have a Type A personality and must consider yourself to be at major risk for atherosclerosis and hypertension. If the answer is equivocal, the possibility of increased risk must be factored in when you determine your overall risk for hypertension and atherosclerosis. If the rest of your pattern suggests low risk, probably nothing further need be done. By contrast, if your overall pattern suggests that you are at increased risk for one or both of these illnesses, then a change in diet as well as a change in behavior may make a big difference.

Table 1 is a list of objective phrases that can be used to determine if you have a Type A personality.

TABLE 1

Things go wrong *more than once a week*

Usually the first finished eating

Spouse or friend *often* told you that you eat too fast

Frequently feel like hurrying someone who takes too long to come to point

Frequently put words in his mouth

Often hurry when plenty of time

Very impatient if have to wait in line

People *definitely agree* you're easily irritated

People *definitely agree* you tend to hurry

Fiery temper when younger

Strong temper nowadays

Really irritated by interruptions

Definitely hard-driving and competitive when younger

Definitely hard-driving and competitive nowadays

Spouse rates *definitely hard-driving and competitive*

Spouse rates generally *too active*

People *definitely agree* you take work too seriously

People *definitely disagree* you have less energy than most

People *definitely agree* you tend to hurry

People *definitely agree* you enjoy competition

Put forth *much more effort* than average at job

Much more responsible than average worker

Hurry *much more of the time* than average worker

Much more precise than average worker
Approach life *much more seriously* than average

Cigarette Smoking

If you smoke cigarettes, you are at increased risk for such diseases as emphysema (a form of chronic lung disease), coronary artery disease, and cancer of the lung. Emphysema is directly caused by cigarette smoking, and no diet will prevent it or lessen its impact. By contrast, cigarette smoking is only one of several major risk factors for atherosclerosis and coronary artery disease. Therefore, if you smoke it is particularly important to minimize any other risk. If your diet is high in saturated fat and cholesterol, this also increases your risk for atherosclerosis by increasing your blood-fat levels. The two risks (smoking and increased blood-fat levels) are additive. Thus, changing your diet may put you into a lower-risk group.

If you smoke, obviously it is desirable to stop or cut back as much as possible. In fact, if you can accomplish this, you may not have to do anything else. If you can't then you must take extra measures to minimize any other risk factors. In the case of lung cancer, although more studies need to be done, there is some evidence that eating a diet rich in vitamin A may afford some protection. Clearly, if you smoke you need all the protection you can get! For you, it is doubly important to choose a diet that is naturally high in vitamin A.

Alcohol

Heavy alcohol consumption unfortunately is a part of the life-style of many Americans. We know that alcohol can be directly toxic to the liver and brain; it can result in severe, even life-threatening illnesses such as cirrhosis or dementia. What heavy users of alcohol often overlook is that they are in a *high-risk group* for certain nutritional disorders. The person who consumes three or more "hard drinks" per day over a prolonged period of time is more likely to suffer from a variety of vitamin and mineral deficiencies than the individual who drinks more moderately or who consumes little or no alcohol, because alcohol interferes specifically with the body's absorption of such vitamins as folic acid, thiamine (vitamin B_1), and pyridoxine (vitamin B_6), and with the absorption of such minerals as zinc and magnesium. Thus, a deficiency of any one or a combination of these nutrients may occur. So heavy drinkers should consume a diet that is high in these nutrients.

Drugs

The use of a variety of drugs is so common that it has become part of the life-style of many Americans. Analgesics, tranquilizers, pills to put you to sleep or keep you awake are consumed by the millions. Some of these drugs will increase your risk for certain nutritional deficiencies. For example, aspirin can cause gastric irritations and microscopic bleeding, which can lead to the loss of enough iron to cause deficiency. Also extremely important in this respect is the contraceptive pill, which can interfere with the absorption of such nutrients as folic acid and vitamin B_6 (pyridoxine). Some women who have been taking oral contraceptives for a long time may be at increased risk for deficiency of these two vitamins. Since alcohol also interferes with the absorption of folic acid and vitamin B_6, heavy drinkers who are on the pill are at double risk. Finally, certain drugs can increase your risk not for nutrient deficiencies but for nutrient excess. Of particular concern is sodium, present in many over-the-counter as well as prescription medications. With the sodium you already get in your diet, this significant extra source can place you in a high-risk category for high blood pressure (hypertension).

Exercise

Until recently our increased standard of living has been accompanied by a decline in physical activity. As more machines have been introduced in our lives, less physical exercise has been exerted. Our society has slowly been transformed from a highly active, physical one to a much more sedentary type. Certainly the policeman on the beat, the firefighter, the construction worker, the farmer all still lead lives full of physical activity, but for many of us, so-called white-collar workers, life means driving to work, taking the elevator to the office, sitting in a chair most of the day, getting back in the car, driving home, and sitting in front of a TV set or reading a book until it is time to retire—not much activity in our routine day-to-day chores. This reduction in physical activity has placed many of us at increased risk for a number of diseases, some of which are nutritionally related. The most important are obesity, atherosclerosis, hypertension, and osteoporosis.

The realization that fitness cannot only increase a person's longevity, but also increase the quality of life and a sense of well-being has led to a revolution in physical activity in the past few years. Jogging, walking, bicycle riding, swimming, health clubs, aerobic dancing, and calisthenics have become part of the life-style of many people. To the extent that we engage in increased physical activity, this reduces our risk for the diseases mentioned above. But don't be fooled; exercise is not the answer to all our problems.

Obesity, atherosclerosis, hypertension, and osteoporosis are all caused by a number of factors acting simultaneously, of which lack of exercise is just one. Depending on how active you are, an increase in physical activity may lower your risk for these diseases. Usually, however, this change in your life-style must be accompanied by other changes, including changes in your diet, if you are to derive maximum benefit.

One word of caution: don't go from being someone who watches Wimbledon on television to a three-set singles player in one step. Begin gradually and work your way slowly into a more active life-style. If you already suffer from one of the above mentioned diseases, increase your exercise under a doctor's supervision. And stick with it! Remember, it is a change in life-style you are seeking, not a short-term change to achieve a defined goal, such as losing five pounds before some important social function. For most of us, increasing physical activity will have positive health benefits. And remember, for some of us, it will reduce our risk for four of the most important diseases prevalent in our society.

How do you decide whether you are too sedentary and need to increase your physical activity? Some sophisticated tests using extremely complicated and expensive equipment can do this very accurately. And in some cases your doctor will want to have these tests done. However, you yourself can make a rough determination by answering a few questions honestly. First, does your job demand a great deal of physical activity, a moderate amount, or little or none? If the answer is a great deal, you need not probe further. Further increasing your physical activity will probably have little effect on reducing your risk. If your answer is little or none, do you indulge in any *regular* form of exercise? For example, do you walk or ride a bike to work, jog daily, play tennis three times a week, swim often? If not, you are a person of low physical activity and your risk for the four diseases mentioned is increased, but you can lower that risk by increasing physical activity. Many people's answers will put them in a category somewhere in between. If you are one of these, you are probably at somewhat increased risk and will probably benefit by increasing your *regular* physical activity. Remember, if you decide that you need to or want to increase your physical activity, pick a form of exercise that you enjoy. Don't jog just because your friends do, if jogging bores you. There are enough ways to increase physical activity to satisfy everyone; pick one you enjoy, get into it gradually, and stick with it. Remember, it is a change in life-style, and life is a long time.

Excessive Dieting

Calorie counting has become an integral part of life for many of us. Every week some magazines tell us about a new way to reduce. A diet book of some sort is a constant fixture on the best-seller list. For the most part, Americans don't diet to cure obesity or to prevent it. They diet to achieve an image that has been equated with good health, youth, fitness, sexiness, beauty, and glamour. And Americans diet not for health reasons primarily, but for cosmetic reasons. Dieting means fewer calories; fewer calories usually mean less food; less food often means fewer nutrients, which in certain susceptible groups can lead to nutrient deficiencies. For example, we have seen that iron is a crucial nutrient, particularly for women. If you are consuming fewer than 1,200 calories per day (many diets restrict calories to even lower levels), you will almost certainly be unable to fulfill your iron requirement. Thus, simply reducing your caloric intake to 1,200 or less will increase your risk for a number of nutrient deficiencies (for example, iron, zinc, vitamin B_6, and folic acid). The situation would be bad enough even if calories were always lowered in a manner that favors the consumption of foods rich in these nutrients. Often, however, this is not the case. Many diets currently used by many people reduce calories by offering a "miracle" program that emphasizes one particular food or type of food. The grapefruit diet, the pineapple diet, the diet that allows mainly meat, the one that allows no meat, the fruit diet, or the high-fat diet are all so restrictive that nutrient deficiencies can and do occur. In most cases the human body with its amazing resiliency is able to recover. In some cases deficiencies of one or more nutrients will occur. In a few cases serious diseases and even death have ensued.

Nutrient deficiencies are not the only problem with the use of unbalanced weight-reduction schemes. Nutrient excesses are equally dangerous. As we shall see, a risk factor for atherosclerosis and for certain cancers is a diet high in fat. There are reducing diets being advocated by a variety of "experts," and followed by millions of people, that are extremely high in fat. These diets are dangerous for us all and particularly so for people who are at high risk for atherosclerosis, cancer of the breast, and cancer of the colon.

If your life is one of constant dieting, ask yourself if you are doing it to treat or prevent obesity. If the answer is yes, then use a balanced reduction in calories that you can sustain for the rest of your life (see Chapter 4). If the answer is no, then stop dieting if you can, or if you must diet, use a low-calorie regime that provides the maximum variety of foods. Avoid the crash programs that promise instant results. Like everything else, even if these programs are successful, there is a price to pay. In this case the price may be too high: increasing your risk for certain serious diseases later in life.

I hope it is clear now that your risk for certain important nutritionally related diseases may depend in great part on your life-style. As you assess your own risk, you must honestly evaluate your living habits. Do you have a Type A personality? Do you smoke, drink to excess, use certain kinds of drugs? Is your level of physical activity low? Are you constantly dieting, and if so, do you use a balanced or an unbalanced approach to weight loss? As we discuss each disease in which nutrition plays an important role, we shall point out which of these practices (if any) increases risk, and how you can lower that risk by either altering your habits, changing your diet, or both.

Your Dietary Pattern

The last, and in some ways the most important, factor in determining your risk for a nutritionally related disease is the kind of dietary pattern you maintain. I am not talking about what you ate during the past twenty-four hours or seven days. I am not talking in terms of weeks or even months. I am talking about your pattern or patterns over the years. Before you can make a rational decision about whether you should change your eating habits, it is important to determine the nature of the diet you actually consume. Is it high in calories, fat, cholesterol, salt? Is it low in fiber, calcium, iron, folic acid? Obviously, if you are at high risk for atherosclerosis, reducing the total and saturated fat and cholesterol will reduce your risk only if your present diet is high in these nutrients. Similarly, increasing the calcium content of what you eat will help lower your risk for osteoporosis only if your diet is low in calcium to begin with.

In each of the following chapters I will be discussing dietary patterns that can lower your risk for certain diseases. Compare these patterns with the way you now eat. For most of you, the differences will be great and your risk will be lowered by instituting a change. For some of you, the differences will be small. If this is the case, you cannot expect major benefits from changing your diet. You will do better to address some of the other risk factors under your control such as the life-style factors discussed in the preceding section. Remember, changing your diet can have a major impact on lowering your risk for certain important diseases, but only if you are already at high risk for them and if you are eating the types of foods that are themselves risk factors for the particular disease. Table 2 is a list of various diseases and the diet that increases risk. In discussing each disease, foods high or low in the offending nutrient will be identified. By comparing your long-

TABLE 2

Disease	Type of diet that increases risk
Atherosclerosis	High fat, high saturated fat, high cholesterol
High blood pressure	High sodium, low calcium(?)
Cancer of the colon and breast	High fat
Diabetes	High calorie
Obesity	High calorie
Dental caries	High refined sugar
Osteoporosis	Low calcium
Anemia	Low iron, low folic acid, low vitamin B_{12}
Constipation-diverticulosis	Low fiber

term dietary pattern with the listed foods, you should be able to assess whether you are increasing your risk and, consequently, whether a dietary change will be beneficial for you.

Scoring Your Risk Potential

We have considered the major risk factors in the most important nutritionally related diseases. They are:

Sex

Race

Family history

Life-style

Present dietary pattern

The importance of each risk factor varies with the specific disease. For example, race is important in high blood pressure, while it is less important in osteoporosis. By contrast, sex is very important in osteoporosis and much less important in high blood pressure. Family history is extremely important in determining risk for obesity, atherosclerosis, high blood pressure, and diabetes, and not very important in determining risk for cancer of the colon or diverticulosis. Life-style is important in atherosclerosis, hypertension, and vitamin and mineral deficiencies, and of little or no importance in cancer of the breast or colon.

We shall also see how different components of your life-style may be particularly important in determining your risk for certain diseases. Smoking is a *major* risk factor in atherosclerosis, a *minor* risk factor in hypertension, and not at all a risk factor in obesity. A Type A personality is an important risk factor in atherosclerosis and hypertension, but it is unimportant in cancer of the breast or colon. Thus, these various components will have a different weight in determining risk for each disease discussed.

Finally, although dietary pattern is an important risk factor in all these diseases, your personal pattern may or may not be contributing to your risk for one or more of them. For these reasons, your risk must be assessed separately for each disease. As you read each chapter you will see that I have assigned a number to each risk factor for the disease under discussion. The numbers will vary with the disease. Below a certain score you are at *low* risk. Above a certain score you are at *high* risk. In between these numbers, your risk is moderate. In each chapter a chart lists the risk factors and their point value. These charts will help you quantitate your risk and give you a written record of your present risk; and it is also a way of scoring any changes that result from your efforts to lower that risk. By no means is it an exact set of numbers to derive an accurate figure for calculating your precise chances of having any specific disease.

In some cases, risk factors are better defined than in others and therefore will carry more weight. All these considerations will be carefully discussed in the chapters that follow. At this point, it is important to note that once you have worked out your risk score for any of the diseases in question you will be able to decide whether a change in diet is appropriate for you. Your decision will not be based on exact, quantitative data. I wish it could be. However, it *will* be based on personal data and therefore will be much more applicable to you than any pronouncements by the government or other groups about benefits to "the American people" in general.

Changing Your Diet

Now that you have determined your risk status and have decided to alter your diet, it is reasonable to ask—how do I know I have reduced my risk? Have I made myself immune to atherosclerosis or hypertension or osteoporosis? I wish there were precise tests which could tell you that your risk has dropped from one level to another. There aren't. I also wish a change in diet could make you immune. It can't. This is where prevention of a nutritional disease becomes much more difficult and complicated than prevention of an infectious disease. When someone has been vaccinated, we can measure within a short time whether the vaccination has taken. There will be antibodies in the blood or a positive skin reaction. Once we are sure that you have been successfully vaccinated against a disease, we can assure you that if you obtain booster shots when necessary, you will not get that disease, you will be immune!

With nutritional diseases there are no antibodies in the blood and there are no guarantees of immunity. People die of heart attacks every day who were in low-risk categories. And conversely, people in high-risk categories live to ripe old ages and die quietly in bed. What you will accomplish by altering your diet is changing the odds. In some cases there will be some tangible evidence that the odds have changed. The level of cholesterol and other blood lipids (fats) will change, or your blood pressure will drop slightly, or you will lose a certain number of pounds. In other cases you will see no change and your doctor will not be able to measure a change. For example, if you decide to go on a low-fat, high-fiber diet to reduce your risk for certain cancers, no *direct* measurement can be made which will tell you that you have accomplished your goal. We can only say that in populations who have changed their dietary patterns in a similar manner, the incidence of these cancers has dropped. In other words, fewer people get cancer of the colon or of the breast if they consume a low-fat diet. In some ways, it's like deciding to wear seat belts. There is no guarantee that you will survive a crash, but the statistics suggest that your chances of survival are better.

A decision to change your diet is a personal one and only you can make that decision. All I can do in the succeeding chapters is to give you the available information to help you make the most informed choices possible. For each disease discussed, the amount of available data will differ. For example, if you reduce the amount of total fat, saturated fat, and cholesterol in your diet, we anticipate that the level of cholesterol in your blood might drop between 15 and 20 percent. If this actually occurs, depending on actual blood levels, we could give you a statistical idea of what your chances are for having a heart attack in the next ten years and to what degree you have lowered your risk. For heart disease we can at least predict the odds with some accuracy. For other diseases our ability to predict is much more limited. For example, we know that consuming adequate amounts of calcium in your younger years will offer some protection from osteoporosis and the brittle bones of later years. However, we don't know how much protection is afforded, and we have no way of monitoring the impact of the dietary change. For osteoporosis then, your decision to change your diet will have to be based on less quantitative data.

Another question that has no doubt already occurred

to you is, when do I have to institute the dietary change to get the maximum benefit? In some cases the peak incidence of the disease you are trying to prevent may be forty to fifty years away. Do you have to change your diet now, or can you wait another ten or twenty years? Again, for many diseases a precise answer will be unavailable. For the most part, however, the earlier you institute the dietary modification, the better your chances for reducing risk. The effects of an improper diet are often cumulative, so that the longer you continue to consume such foods, the harder it will be to overcome your risk.

At this point it may seem that the potential benefits are not worth the long-term commitment. Not true. We are about to discuss some of the most serious diseases that afflict our society. These diseases occur not in one person in a million or in one in a thousand, but cumulatively in *one out of every two individuals*. It is at least even money that you will eventually suffer from one or more of these diseases. If a dietary change can significantly lower your risk for one or more of them, especially if this can be accomplished while still allowing you a wide variety of food choices, isn't it worth at least trying to make such a change?

Chapter 2

Atherosclerosis

Atherosclerosis (hardening of the arteries) is a process that develops early in life and progresses as an individual gets older. Fatty materials known as lipids, carried in the blood mainly in the form of cholesterol, are deposited in the lining of arteries and form rough plaques that slowly increase in size. This process gradually reduces the opening in the artery through which blood can flow. Eventually the artery can become completely blocked, cutting off the blood supply to the areas it usually feeds. If the artery (coronary artery) cannot bring blood to the heart tissue the person suffers a heart attack. If the clogged artery services a portion of the brain, a stroke will follow. Thus, a heart attack or a stroke is not a primary disease of the heart or brain, but a disease of the blood vessels that supply these organs. In addition to such dramatic consequences of atherosclerosis as heart attack or stroke, more insidious consequences may occur. Perhaps the most serious is senility, which is believed to be caused by a gradual hardening of many of the smaller arteries to the brain, which in turn causes a generalized reduction in the flow of blood to that organ. The result is confusion, loss of memory, and, finally, incoherence.

Atherosclerosis is a disease of man. It does not occur under natural conditions in any other animal, and even under controlled laboratory conditions, very few animals can be induced to develop the disease. In part, atherosclerosis can be blamed on a person's genes. It definitely runs in families. But for most of us, genes are not as important as the way we live. If any disease can be blamed specifically on life-style, it is atherosclerosis. The disease is almost unheard of in primitive societies. Yet it is the scourge of the western world. Eliminating atherosclerosis would easily add ten years to people's average life expectancy, and immensely improve the quality of life for millions.

What then is the cause of this important disease? There is no one cause; there are many. Some we know about; about others, we do not. All of them are related either directly or indirectly to life-style or diet. Since there is no single cause of atherosclerosis, we must talk instead about risk factors. The major risk factors for developing atherosclerosis are:

Type A personality

Cigarette smoking

Hyperlipidemia (high blood-fat levels), particularly high
    blood-cholesterol levels

Hypertension (high blood pressure)

Diabetes

Are You at Risk for Atherosclerosis?

The presence of any one of the above factors is all that is necessary to place you at risk for atherosclerosis. Thus, if you put down five points each for Type A personality, cigarette smoking, hyperlipidemia, hypertension, and diabetes, a score of 5 or greater puts you in a high-risk category. In addition, there are several other factors which increase your risk. If you are male, add one more point, since men seem to be slightly more at risk for atherosclerosis than women, independent of the major risk factors. If you have a strong family history, add two points; if you are obese, add two points, since obesity increases your chances of developing hyperlipidemia, hypertension, and diabetes, conditions which can lead to atherosclerosis. Thus, an obese male with a strong family history can be in a high-risk category for atherosclerosis without having any of the major risk factors listed. You should be able to determine with a good deal of certainty whether you have some of these risk factors. For the other factors, it may be much more difficult to be sure and assign a number to them.

Let us use a hypothetical example. You are male (one point), you don't smoke (zero points), your blood pressure is a normal 120/80 (zero points), and you don't have diabetes (zero points). The risk factors are easily scored. You are either male or female; you either smoke or don't smoke; your blood pressure is either high or normal; and you either do or do not have diabetes. The other risk factors are not so simple to assess. Do you have a Type A personality? Let your spouse or a close friend decide whether you are extremely hard driving, constantly under pressure, always harried by deadlines, and whether the type of job you have exacerbates these traits.

Score the categories on page 42 as honestly as you can. For some of you, if the answer is definitely yes, score 5; for others, if it is definitely no, score 0. Many of you will not be sure how to answer. Score yourself between 1 and 4 as best you can. If you are going to err, err on the high side.

Do you have a positive family history? Draw your family health tree. If several close relatives definitely had or suffer from atherosclerosis, heart attack, stroke, or were known or are known to have hyperlipidemia (high blood-fat or cholesterol levels), score 2. If no relatives or only a few distant ones have had any of these problems, score

0. If your family history puts you in a category in between, score 1.

Are you obese? We will discuss obesity and its prevention and treatment in Chapter 4. For our present purposes, if you are 20 percent above your ideal weight this gives you a score of 2; 10 percent above, a score of 1; and below your ideal weight, a score of 0 (see the tables on page 77).

Do you have hyperlipidemia? Even though blood levels of cholesterol and other lipids (fats) can be measured very accurately, the answer to this question is not simple.

Hyperlipidemia means high blood levels of lipids or fats. The most important of these blood fats is cholesterol. The higher your blood levels of cholesterol, the greater your chances of developing atherosclerosis. We often hear that the normal blood-cholesterol level is around 250 milligrams (mg) per 100 milliliters (ml), but this is really not correct. The average level in the middle-aged population in the United States may be as high as that but only because we are a population that consumes a diet that results in high levels of blood cholesterol. That this is our average does not make it normal. In certain populations who do not consume such a diet, the average level is about 175 mg per 100 ml. Since the risk for developing atherosclerosis increases the higher your blood cholesterol levels are (particularly when these levels are above 200 mg per 100 ml), it is my belief that we should strive for levels below 200 mg, and that only people who maintain these levels should be considered as having normal levels. By using a criterion of 175 mg per 100 ml as normal, the majority of people in our society will have high cholesterol levels. This phenomenon is related to our life-style and can be changed by altering our diet.

Is your serum cholesterol too high? You don't know? The first step in reducing your risk for atherosclerosis is to find out. Most physicians will order a blood cholesterol level test as part of a routine physical. If your doctor does not, tell him to. And get the result—not whether the level is normal or not, but the actual number. If your level is over 175 mg per 100 ml, give yourself a score of 1; if it is above 185, score 2; if it is 200, score 3; if 225, score 4; and if 250, score 5. To understand fully why these values for serum cholesterol are so important, we must examine what controls the level of cholesterol in our blood.

Cholesterol is manufactured in the body and is also present in the diet. The level in the blood is determined by the availability from these two sources. Most of the body's cholesterol is made in the liver. From there, it is transported to other organs that need it. For example, many of the hormones manufactured in the adrenal gland are made from cholesterol; the insulation around nerve sheaths in the brain is mostly cholesterol; the gall bladder uses cholesterol in the production of bile used in digestion. Cholesterol is so important that it is reabsorbed from bile secreted into the intestines. Cholesterol is essential for life; only when it is present in excess amounts is it dangerous. Your body knows this and tries to keep the level of cholesterol constant. If too much is consumed in the diet, the body makes less. However, this protective mechanism can be overwhelmed if we consume very large quantities of cholesterol or saturated fat. These *saturated* fats, found mainly in meat and dairy products, will raise the level of blood cholesterol just as will dietary cholesterol itself. By contrast, *polyunsaturated* fats in our diet, obtained largely from vegetable sources, are believed to lower blood-cholesterol levels. Exactly how these different types of fats influence the levels of blood cholesterol is not known. A good way to remember which kind of fat is which is that saturated fats are usually hard, whereas polyunsaturated fats are usually soft or liquid.

Cholesterol is transported in the blood attached to protein carriers of different sizes, forming lipoproteins. Most cholesterol is carried by a light (low-density) lipoprotein, or LDL, and it is the amount of cholesterol carried in this form which concerns us most and which is most sensitive to dietary saturated fat and cholesterol. High levels of total serum cholesterol almost always mean high levels of LDL cholesterol. A small amount of cholesterol is carried by another protein which is of much higher density and hence is called high-density lipoprotein, or HDL. This form of cholesterol is desirable, and the higher amounts the better, because it is believed that this cholesterol actually comes from arterial plaques and thus reduces the amount of atherosclerosis present. A level of HDL cholesterol *above* 45 mg per 100 ml reduces your risk for atherosclerosis. Thus, if you know your HDL levels, you can score more accurately: if they are above 45 mg, *subtract* one point; if from 40 to 45 mg, add zero; and if below 40 mg, add one point.

Your Atherosclerosis Score

Now you are ready to add up your score. Fill in the chart below.

Risk Factor	Maximum Score	Your Score
Sex	1 (male)	
Family history	2	
Type A personality	5	
Cigarette smoking	5	
Hyperlipidemia	6	
Hypertension	5	
Diabetes	5	
Obesity	2	
Total	31	

After you have added up your score, a look at the following chart will indicate your risk:

Below 5	low risk
5–9	moderate risk
10–19	high risk
20 and above	very high risk

If your score is below 5, you can skip the rest of this chapter and move on to the next chapter. (You may want to read it anyway, just so you can advise a friend or relative.)

If your score is 5 or above, you should take measures to lower it. Each of the risk factors should be approached separately. Obviously you can't change your sex or your family history. Changing your personality or your job may be extremely difficult. If you smoke, your high score should provide some incentive to stop. High blood pressure must be treated by a physician and may require drugs and dietary therapy (see Chapter 3). If you are obese, you should definitely attempt weight reduction (see Chapter 4). Diabetes is a serious disease and must also be managed by a doctor. This treatment may entail the use of insulin and careful attention to your diet. Finally, if you have hyperlipidemia, specific dietary treatment is required.

Do You Need to Modify Your Diet?

For those of you who have scores of 5 or higher, the chances are very good that dietary modification will be helpful. The next step is to examine the components of your score more carefully.

Focus on your hyperlipidemia score. If it is 3 or more, then a modified-fat diet should help lower your risk for atherosclerosis no matter the source of the other points. If your hyperlipidemia score is 2 or less (serum-cholesterol level of under 200), and the only other risk factors are having a Type A personality or cigarette smoking, you will benefit much more by eliminating these factors than by changing your diet. If your other points are coming from the other risk factors—that is, from family history, hypertension, diabetes, or obesity—you should use the modified-fat diet in addition to specific means aimed at eliminating the particular risk factor. The chart below indicates who should use and who does not need to use a modified-fat diet:

Total score below 5—	not necessary.
Total score 5 and above—	hyperlipidemia score 3 and above—everyone.
Total score 5 and above—	hyperlipidemia score 2 and below—remaining points from Type A personality and cigarette smoking. Not necessary (if you can eliminate these risk factors).
Total score 5 and above—	hyperlipidemia score 2 and below—remaining points from risk factors other than Type A personality and cigarette smoking—everyone.

Remember, now that you have determined your risk and decided whether or not a modified-fat diet can help you lower that risk, you must still address the other risk factors directly because the major ones listed on page 42 are additive. That is, if you are a smoker who has hyperlipidemia, you are at greater risk than if you had either risk factor alone. Hypertension or diabetes will each elevate that risk. This is the reason for using the atherosclerosis scoring system that I have outlined. Obviously unless you deal with each risk factor, your chances of getting atherosclerosis will be higher. In this chapter I will discuss only the modified-fat diet since it is the one that has a direct impact on atherosclerosis. If you have hypertension, diabetes, or obesity, you are at risk for other diseases in addition to atherosclerosis. In each of these conditions, other dietary modifications may be necessary in addition to the modified-fat diet discussed here. These modifications will be described in the appropriate chapters.

Dietary Principles to Follow

Once you have decided to consume a diet aimed at lowering your risk for atherosclerosis, the guidelines are quite simple to follow. They have been developed from numerous experimental studies and also by simply imitating the diets of groups of people who have the lowest incidence of coronary artery disease. One of the earliest projects to identify diet change as a successful means of lowering blood cholesterol was devised by the Anti-Coronary Club of the Bureau of Nutrition, New York City Department of Health. Doctor Norman Jolliffe, the project's director, coined its name, "the Prudent Diet."

This diet is designed to lower your blood cholesterol by modifying one nutrient—FAT. To dine the "Prudent" way, you should limit the amount and the kinds of fat you eat. By amount, I mean that fat should contribute no more than one-third of your total dietary calories. (The rest of the calories should come from starches, sugars, and protein.) By kinds of fat I mean that the diet should contain at least as much polyunsaturated fat as saturated fat. In addition, your cholesterol intake should be kept under 300 mg per day. To understand these guidelines, let us take a closer look at foods.

All foods are derived from either animal or plant sources. Those from animal sources include all red meat, poultry, fish, shellfish, eggs, milk, cheese, and other products derived from these foods. Those from plant sources include fruits, vegetables, grains, beans, and nuts.

Foods from Animal Sources
Cholesterol, a waxy fat, is a vital compound found in all animals but not in plants. The amount of cholesterol

present varies among meats and other foods from animal sources. The greatest concentration of cholesterol is found in eggs and organ meats (such as beef, calves liver, or chicken livers, kidneys, heart, brains, and fish roe). Table 3 lists the approximate cholesterol content of common

Table 3   Average Cholesterol Content of Common Meats

Food	mg Cholesterol
1. Liver (3 oz.)	372
2. Egg (large)	252
3. Shrimp, canned (3 oz.)	128
4. Veal (3 oz.)	86
5. Lamb (3 oz.)	83
6. Beef (3 oz.)	80
7. Pork (3 oz.)	76
8. Lobster (3 oz.)	72
9. Chicken (½ breast, no skin)	63
10. Clams, canned (½ cup)	50
11. Chicken (1 drumstick)	39
12. Fish, fillet (3 oz.)	34–75

meats. It is important to note that the more fat present on the meat, the greater the amount of cholesterol. Therefore, the rule is: meat must be lean and well trimmed. Because some meats can never be lean and trimmed enough, they are not recommended for regular consumption. Table 4 lists those high-fat meats as well as recommended lean cuts.

Food from Plant Sources

Fruits, vegetables, grains, and grain products (such as breads, pastas, breakfast cereals, rice, etc.) and beans are virtually fat-free. Since the amount of fat these foods contain is nil, the kind of fat is not a problem. Remember, we are talking here of food as it is grown. If during preparation fat (such as butter or margarine) is used, you should determine how much and what kind was added.

TABLE 4 Recommended and Prohibited Meats for the Prudent Diet

Recommended	Prohibited
All fish	Duck
All shellfish	Goose
Veal, all cuts	Cold cuts
Chicken fryers & broilers*	Frankfurters
Rock Cornish hen*	Sausage
Turkey (not self-basting)*	
	Beef:
Beef:	Shell strip
Bottom round	T-bone steak
Top round	Club steak
Eye round	Sirloin
Sirloin tip	Chuck
Roast filet	Rib roast
Rump	Shoulder roast
Bottom round	Porterhouse steak
Ground round	Brisket
Flank steak	Short ribs
Minute or cubed steak	Tongue
Lamb:	Lamb:
Roast leg of lamb	Shanks
Lamb steaks	Loin lamb chops
	Rib chops
Pork:	Lamb stew
Lean cured ham	
Lean ham steak	Pork:
	Loin pork chops
	Roast loin of pork
	Canadian bacon
	Bacon
	Spareribs
	Salt pork
	Ham hocks

*without skin

There is a group of plant products that is very important in the Prudent Diet: seeds, nuts, and the fats derived from plant sources. The most familiar products in this group are vegetable oils and margarines made from them. In choosing these foods, it is important to differentiate between kinds of fats.

There are three basic kinds of fats in nature: the saturated fats (SF), the monounsaturated fats (MF), and the polyunsaturated fats (PF). The three fats differ in chemical structure: the SF are typically solid, the PF are liquid, and the MF are roughly in between. There are several varieties of each kind of fat, but no fat is pure SF, MF, or PF; that is, all fats are a natural mixture of all three. Some fats—lard, for example—are composed almost entirely of SF. Corn oil is approximately four parts PF, two parts MF, and one part SF. Nutritionists describe a fat by the amount of PF compared with the amount of SF, or more simply, by its "P:S ratio." You can say, then, that corn oil has a P:S ratio of 4:1. (Monounsaturated fats are "neutral" and are not a part of the ratio.)

The idea in the Prudent Diet is to use those fats that are high in PF and low in SF (that is, those that have a high P:S ratio) and limit those fats and foods that are low in PF and high in SF (or those with a low P:S ratio). Table 5 lists foods and their predominant kinds of fats. Remember, the harder or more solid a fat is, the more saturated it is; we can therefore correctly deduce that the soft margarines have a higher P:S ratio than the stick margarines.

By the way, the fats in meats, poultry, and dairy products also contain small amounts of polyunsaturated fat. The amount varies with each animal. For example, beef fat has an average P:S ratio of 1:18; pork has a ratio of 1:4, and chicken and fish have a ratio of 1:1.

TABLE 5   Distribution of Fats in Common Foods

High in Polyunsaturated Fats

Safflower oil	Soybeans
Corn oil	Sunflower seeds
Soft margarine: made of corn oil	Sesame seeds
Walnuts	Oils made from these seeds

Moderately High in Polyunsaturated Fats

Soybean oil	Commercial salad dressings
Cottonseed oil	Mayonnaise
Other soft margarines	

High in Monounsaturated fats

Peanut oil	Pecans
Peanuts and peanut butter	Cashews
Olive oil	Brazil nuts
Olives	Avocados
Almonds	

High in Saturated Fats

Meats high in fat: sausages, cold cuts, prime cuts, etc.	Stick margarines
Chicken fat	Coconut oil
Meat drippings	Butter and products with dairy fat, for example, cheese, cream, whole milk, ice cream, chocolate, bakery items
Lard	
Hydrogenated shortening	

High in Cholesterol

Egg yolks	Pâté
Liver	Caviar
Kidneys	Dairy products
Sweetbreads	Products made with the above, for example, cakes, pies, pastries, gravies, etc.
Brains	
Heart	

At the Table

Now we must arrange all this information into some eating suggestions. In order to limit the total amount of fat and cholesterol, we must limit the main sources of these substances—the animal products in our diet. The maximum amount of meat (this means *anything* with fins, fur, or feathers) to be eaten per day is six ounces if your total intake of calories is under 1,500, and eight ounces if your total intake exceeds 1,500 calories. This level ensures a cholesterol intake that will be less than 300 mg per day. At the same time it limits the amount of fat being contributed by primarily high-saturated-fat (or low P:S ratio) foods. Red meat (beef, lamb, and pork) should be limited to sixteen ounces per week.

To these amounts you must add three tablespoons of a high polyunsaturated fat per day (for six ounces of meat) or four tablespoons per day (for eight ounces of meat). This amount of fat should include what you use as a spread, what you use in cooking (including frying at home), and what you use on salads. These three or four tablespoons ensure a dietary P:S ratio of 2:1 or higher.

Limit egg yolks to two per week whether eaten plain or in prepared foods. Egg whites can be eaten in unlimited quantities. No additional fat-containing foods (such as those listed in Table 5, page 49) should be eaten.

All other low-fat foods (such as fruits, vegetables, low-fat dairy products, grains, beans, etc.) can be eaten in unlimited quantities unless you are watching your weight. In this case, use your discretion on high-sugar foods. Altogether, the amount of fat from the meat and the added three or four tablespoons of oil will contribute no more than one-third of your total calories.

Desserts should be low in fat. For example, you can eat gelatin, fruit ices, low-fat yogurt, angel-food cake, or homemade products containing the recommended kinds and amounts of fat.

Basically the Prudent Diet is not very different from the way many people eat in many parts of the world—particularly in areas where incidence of heart disease is extremely low. The difference is mainly in the ingredients rather than in foods eaten.

Dining Out

An evening of fine dining as well as a routine lunch hour need not be replaced with the monotonous brown bag just because your food selection requires more attention. You will be surprised at the flexibility the Prudent Diet guidelines offer the seasoned patron of the soup line. Whether at a company cafeteria, a short-order breakfast, or a gourmet feast, you should always heed certain signals. For starters, look for words and phrases which describe the selection in such a way that you know they are high in calories and fat and hence can avoid them. Some of these tempting but dangerous descriptive phrases include:

- "buttery," "buttered," or "butter sauce"
- "sautéed," "fried," "pan-fried," or "crispy"
- "creamed," "cream sauce," or "in its own gravy"
- "au gratin," "Parmesan," "in cheese sauce," or "escalloped"
- "au lait," "à la mode," or "au fromage"
- "marinated," "stewed," "basted," or "en casserole"
- "prime," "hash," "pot pie," and "hollandaise"

On the other hand, the following descriptions are welcome invitations:

- "pickled," "tomato sauce," "steamed," or "in broth"
- "in its own juice," "poached," or "garden-fresh"
- "roasted," "stir-fried," and "cocktail sauce"

Because many dishes and restaurants vary, an easy rule to follow is that the more simply prepared a food is, the lower in fat it is. Spices and seasonings such as garlic, curry, bay leaves, oregano, ginger, onion, and dill, and garnishes like parsley, lemon slices, or pimentos do not contribute any fat to the dish, though they can enhance the flavor and appeal immensely. In general, poultry, fish, and seafood are the best selections because they are naturally low in fat and can be prepared without the addition of saturated fats and still taste delicious. Be aware that many broiled entrées have been basted with butter or olive oil.

Salads offer a tremendous variety of flavors and textures while still permitting you, the diner, utmost control over the kinds and amounts of fat in the meal. It is best to request that dressings be served "on the side" so that you can serve yourself an appropriate amount.

Here is a summary of recommended menu selections:

Appetizers—fresh fruits and vegetables as crudités or juices; seafood cocktail. (Avoid sour or sweet cream and seasoned butter or oils.)

Soups—clear consomme or broth with noodles or vegetables, if desired. (Avoid cheese soups, cream soups, egg soups, and onion soup; bean soups should be fat-free.)

Salads—green and tossed salads; additions may include chicken, turkey, seafood, tuna, lean roast beef, lean ham (as in a chef's salad), clear gelatin molds; cole slaw, potato, and Waldorf salad should have a minimum of mayonnaise. (Avoid cheese and creamy dressings.)

Fish—any variety prepared without fat. (Avoid tartar sauce.)

Poultry—chicken, turkey, Rock Cornish hen, prepared without fat and with skin removed. (Avoid goose and duck, and fried or batter-dipped coatings.)

Red meat—always lean hindquarter cuts of beef, lamb, and

pork; all cuts of veal. (Avoid prime cuts, gravy, breaded coatings, any ground beef; cook as well done as is palatable.)

Fruits—as much as you like. (Avoid cream or whipped toppings.)

Vegetables—if served plain, as much as you like.

Other—beans and peas without oil or sauce; walnuts and sunflower seeds.

Bread—all sandwich bread, breadsticks, hard rolls; French and Italian bread, and Syrian pita; wafers and "toasts." (Avoid biscuits, croissants, corn, bran, and blueberry muffins, butter rolls.)

Desserts—angel-food cake, gelatin desserts, frozen fruit ices, and low-fat frozen dairy products. (Avoid cream and nondairy milk substitutes.)

Beverages—low-fat milk products, carbonated and alcoholic beverages, fruit juices, coffee, and tea. (Avoid cream and nondairy milk substitutes.)

Extras—pickles, relishes, mustard, Worcestershire sauce, catsup, steak sauce, lemon juice, vinegar, spices, and herbs.

How does this sound?

Tomato Juice
Shrimp Cocktail
Tossed Salad
Breadsticks
Veal and Mushrooms
Dilled Carrots with Pearl Onions
Angel-Food Cake with Cherry Sauce
Coffee

When you get a yen for an international treat, Oriental dishes are usually fairly low in fat and what fat is used may be a polyunsaturated oil (like sesame oil, or, at worst, peanut oil) instead of the olive oil so often used in Italian cooking, the butter used in French cooking, or the solid fats so often utilized by American fast-food chains. However, many commercial kitchens, regardless of their ethnic theme, use soybean oil. If soybean or corn oil is used, then you can lift the restriction on fried foods. Do remember that the amount of fat is just as important as the kind; you should not overshoot the recommended amount even if it is the recommended kind.

Alcoholic beverages are not limited in the Prudent Diet because they do not have any effect on the blood cholesterol level. However, excessive intake of alcohol or any other high-calorie food or beverage contributes to body fat, and excess body fat does contribute to elevating the blood cholesterol level.

The "carry-out" breakfast, often eaten by commuters, can be transformed from those infamous offenders—a fried-egg sandwich, a doughnut, or Danish pastry and coffee—to great beginners such as an English muffin or a hard roll with jelly. (Avoid high-fat corn and bran muffins, which are as rich as outlawed doughnuts, and pass up stick margarine or butter.) Another portable breakfast is fresh fruit and low-fat cottage cheese. (Who says that can't also be a standby lunch?)

Snacks during the day can be popcorn, pretzels, dried and fresh fruits and vegetables, low-fat yogurt (frozen or regular), walnuts, or sunflower seeds.

Of course, there are occasions when prudence takes a backseat. But as a routine, keep the guidelines, not the fats, on the top of your tongue, and *enjoy.*

An Extra Added Benefit If you are somewhat overweight, the Prudent Diet is low-calorie even if the portions you eat remain the same size as those you ate before, because the diet is lower in fat, the nutrient with the highest caloric density. Let me illustrate. Suppose your regular diet contained 2,800 calories, and consisted of foods that contained 45 percent of the calories from fat. On the

Prudent Diet you have reduced your fat intake by 15 percent, or 420 calories, and increased your carbohydrate intake by 15 percent, or 200 calories (since carbohydrate contains less than one-half the calories per gram of fat). Thus, you have saved 220 calories per day without limiting the amount of food you eat.

We can look at this in a different way. Suppose you are of normal weight and don't need to lose; you can consume larger portions of the Prudent Diet than you could before in order to use up those 220 calories. Or you can have an extra low-fat snack or two. Or perhaps a glass or two of wine with dinner, a practice which might even help further reduce your risk for atherosclerosis. Thus, whether you are overweight or not, this diet has certain advantages over the more traditional higher-fat diet.

Increasing Your Activity

So far we have spoken of the major way to reduce a high-serum-cholesterol level by consuming the low-total-fat, low-saturated-fat, low-cholesterol, relatively high-polyunsaturated-fat diet sometimes called the Prudent Diet. Is there a way to increase even further our HDL-cholesterol level and thereby lower our risk for atherosclerosis? We already know several ways, and no doubt there are others that have yet to be discovered. Probably the most important thing you can do now to raise your HDL-cholesterol level is to increase your activity.

Several studies have shown that athletes, particularly those engaged in endurance sports, have higher HDL-cholesterol levels than comparable individuals not engaged in these sports. Some data suggest that individuals with low levels of HDL cholesterol can increase these levels by engaging in such activities as walking, jogging, swimming, or bicycle riding. There is no question that cardiovascular fitness can be improved in any sedentary individual who carefully undertakes an exercise program. If you have low levels of HDL cholesterol, you will derive a double benefit from such a fitness program.

Consuming Alcoholic Beverages

When it comes to consuming alcoholic beverages, I have good news and bad news. First the good news. There is evidence that *moderate* alcohol consumption will raise the level of HDL cholesterol. Thus, one martini before dinner, or one or two glasses of wine during dinner, will reduce your risk for atherosclerosis. Perhaps that explains why the death rate from coronary artery disease in France is about one-fifth that in the United States. Now the bad news. Heavy drinking will not only result in its own serious consequences (which may explain why the death rate from cirrhosis of the liver is five times as high in France as in the United States), but it may also lower HDL-cholesterol levels. Thus, a little is good but a lot is not better. The key word with alcohol as far as lowering your risk for atherosclerosis is *moderation.*

Taking Out an Insurance Policy

You may ask, Even though my score is under five, will this kind of life-style change offer me insurance? That is, can it lower my risk for atherosclerosis even if only slightly? This is perhaps the most difficult question to answer because we simply do not have the data available to speak with any conviction. In fact, it is in trying to answer this question that many of the experts disagree. From your own standpoint, there is no evidence that such insurance is of great value, particularly if it inhibits you from making other dietary changes that in your case might be more valuable—for example, a low-calorie diet if you are obese, or a high-calcium diet if you are at risk for osteoporosis or brittle bones. On the other hand, if all Americans began to eat more low-fat, low-cholesterol foods, such a diet would become the norm as it is in many countries rather than the exception as it is in the United States. Such a change in our dietary pattern would undoubtedly lower the incidence of atherosclerosis and its complications. You may not be helping yourself, but you could be part of a movement that will help your neighbors and perhaps even your children. Thus when our government "recommends" that all Americans eat a diet that is lower in total fat and cholesterol, it does so with the full knowledge that although it may be of no benefit to you personally, such a dietary change would be of enormous value to the American public as a whole.

Chapter 3

Hypertension (High Blood Pressure)

The blood circulating through the body generates a certain pressure within the arteries and veins. The heart creates this pressure by forcing the blood out of its chambers, into the main artery or aorta, and through its branches toward the various tissues in the body. Blood pressure within any artery is never constant, but oscillates between a high and a low value depending on whether the heart is contracting or relaxing. During a contraction the blood is forced into the arteries at maximum pressure. We call this the systolic pressure. During the period of relaxation and while the heart is refilling with blood, the pressure within the arteries drops to a lower level; this is called the diastolic pressure. Since contractions last for a relatively short period, the arteries are exposed to the diastolic pressure most of the time. When we take our blood pressure, we get two values, the higher being the systolic pressure and the lower the diastolic pressure. The normal value is around 120/80 millimeters (mm) of mercury (Hg) when the blood pressure is taken in the arm in the normal manner. High blood pressure is a condition in which the systolic pressure reaches a level of 140 or above, or when the diastolic pressure reaches 90 or above. A high diastolic pressure is considered more dangerous because the arteries are exposed to this elevated pressure most of the time. As with any liquid flowing through a pipe, the pressure within the pipe can be increased by narrowing the opening and forcing the same amount of liquid through it. The amount of blood within our system is relatively constant. Hence, if our arteries narrow either by contracting their muscular walls or as a result of some disease process, such as atherosclerosis, the pressure within them increases.

High blood pressure favors the deposition of cholesterol from the blood into the arterial wall; hence, it is a primary risk factor for developing atherosclerosis. In addition, high blood pressure can cause a ballooning (called an aneurism) and an actual rupture of a blood vessel. This latter case often occurs in one of the smaller vessels leading to the brain, causing a cerebral hemorrhage or stroke. Finally, prolonged high blood pressure can damage small vessels in the kidney, leading to scarring of that organ and to kidney failure, and can put a strain on the heart muscle, which can lead to heart failure.

There is no doubt that hypertension is a genetic disease. It is much more common in blacks than in whites in the United States, and in both races it runs in families. But genetics is only one part of the story. In the United States, blood pressure rises with age. Until recently this rise was interpreted as normal; the older a person was, the higher his blood pressure could be and still be considered normal. In other countries, particularly among certain primitive societies, such as Greenland Eskimos, Australian aborigines, Polynesians, African Bushmen, and Amerindians, there is no rise in blood pressure with age. Moreover, within these cultures high blood pressure is virtually nonexistent. By contrast, in the United States the incidence of high blood pressure has been estimated to be as high as 30 percent. In China and Japan it is even higher.

While there are many cultural differences existing between these primitive societies and the United States or China or Japan, the difference that relates to high blood pressure is in the diet. And while there are many differences between the diets of the United States, China, and Japan, the one similarity again relating to hypertension is that they are all high in salt, or more precisely in sodium, a major ingredient of salt.

A study involving a group of Samburu from northern Kenya very clearly illustrates the role of salt in causing high blood pressure. Traditionally these nomads consume a diet of meat and milk which is low in sodium. The study followed a group after it was drafted into the Kenyan army, where the national diet of maize meal and other foods raised the sodium intake of these men fivefold. During the second year of service, their blood pressure began to increase and continued to increase throughout their six years of service.

Knowledge of this relationship between high sodium intake and hypertension is not new. In fact, before the advent of modern drug therapy the only way to control high blood pressure was with a very low-salt diet. Today this approach is rarely used because of the restrictive nature of such a diet and because drugs to control hypertension are so effective. Many of these drugs, however, work by causing the body to eliminate more sodium through the kidneys, thus effectively reducing the amount of salt within the tissues and body fluids.

Although the extremely low-salt diet necessary to *treat* high blood pressure is not practical in *preventing* high blood pressure, recent evidence would suggest that moderate salt reduction may be an effective preventive measure in susceptible populations. Animal studies have not only strengthened this assumption, but have begun to shed light on why this may be true.

As in humans, hypertension in rats is a genetic disease. Only certain strains of rats will develop the disease no matter how much salt they eat. However, even in susceptible strains, high blood pressure appears only when the salt content of the diet is increased. This increase does not need to be dramatic but can be quite moderate. Once hypertension develops, however, returning the animal to its previous diet will not lower its blood pressure. Only *drastically reducing* the salt content of the animal's diet will have any effect. Thus, whereas it takes only a small increase in dietary sodium intake to *produce* hypertension, it takes a very large decrease to *control* it once it has developed.

The same experiments have begun to unravel the mystery of why this moderate salt increase results in hypertension in particular strains of animals. Sodium is an element that is essential for life. It is present in all cells and in all body fluids. The body must therefore regulate the amount of sodium it contains. This regulation takes place primarily through the kidneys. When too little sodium is available, the kidney efficiently reabsorbs it, reducing the amount excreted in the urine. When too much sodium is available, the kidney filters it from the blood and passes it into the urine. In the kidney blood is filtered through a small complex of arteries called the glomerulus. The higher the pressure in these arteries, the more efficient the filtration. In order to filter properly, the kidney has a mechanism to raise and lower blood pressure. This mechanism involves the secretion of certain hormones which cause the arterial walls to contract, thus increasing the pressure of the blood circulating through them. In certain strains of animals, and presumably also in susceptible people, a moderate increase in salt intake will invoke this mechanism. Once the arteries have been contracted for a long time, they become more fixed in that condition and will not relax as easily when salt intake is lowered. Thus, the way in which your genes determine whether you are prone to hypertension is by how well the kidney regulates the level of salt intake through hormonal response. In some people even mild increases in dietary sodium will evoke this response; such people are susceptible to high blood pressure. In other people even large increases in dietary sodium can be handled by the kidney without any increase in blood pressure; such people are resistant to hypertension. As the kidney gets older, its ability to filter becomes less efficient; therefore, it has to raise the blood pressure at lower and lower salt intakes. This is why in a society like ours, which consumes relatively high quantities of sodium, blood pressure rises with age. By contrast, in societies in which people consume small amounts of sodium, kidneys filter more efficiently, even in older people, without raising blood pressure.

A second dietary factor that is related to hypertension concerns the consistent consumption of too many calories, leading to obesity. The more overweight you are, the greater your chances for high blood pressure. This increased risk in overweight people is independent of the amount of sodium in their diet. Thus, at any given sodium intake, an obese individual is more prone to hypertension than a lean individual. If you are susceptible to hypertension, stay lean if you are already thin and lose weight if you are already too heavy. The principles for losing weight or maintaining your ideal weight are discussed in detail in Chapter 4.

Very recent studies in animals have suggested that hypertension may be related to low calcium intake. These studies are just beginning and it is too early to tell whether they will have any significance for humans. The American diet tends to be low in calcium, and there are good reasons why increasing the amount of dietary calcium may be beneficial. Prevention of hypertension may add one more important reason.

In this chapter we are focusing on the *prevention* of high blood pressure, not its *treatment*. If we wish to prevent this or any illness, we either must institute preventive measures in the entire population or we must be able to identify those who are most *at risk* and institute these measures in that group only. Americans consume far more salt than they need to. So there is no reason why the entire population could not lower its salt intake. This, in fact, is what is being recommended by several government bodies. While on the surface this recommendation may sound reasonable, it is an oversimplification that may not achieve its desired end even if most people adopt it. The reason is that for those people who are not at risk, slightly lowering their salt intake is unnecessary. By contrast, for those people who are at high risk, a slight lowering may not be enough. What is necessary then is to identify people at high risk for hypertension and for those people to limit their sodium intake sufficiently to prevent high blood pressure. Unfortunately, we are not able to identify all people at risk; and even for those whom we can identify, the precise amount of salt they can safely consume is unknown. However, we are doing much better in both these areas than we were just a few years ago. While we have no foolproof method, it is now possible at least to identify many people at risk before their blood pressure actually rises.

How then do you know if you are at risk for high blood pressure?

First—do you know what your blood pressure is? You should have it taken every year, preferably every six months. You don't need to see a physician for this. There are machines in public places, free clinics, and home-use machines. If your blood pressure is 120/80 or lower, it is normal. If the systolic pressure is over 140, or the diastolic pressure is over 90, you have high blood pressure and should seek medical advice. If your systolic reading is consistently between 120 and 140, or if your diastolic reading is between 85 and 90, you are at risk and preventive measures are indicated.

Second—are you overweight? If the scales indicate you are 10 percent overweight or more, your risk for hypertension is increased and weight loss is indicated.

Third—is there a family history of hypertension or a clear

familial tendency toward higher blood pressure? This may require some detective work. Trace back as far as you can; ask your relatives what they can remember. Did anyone die of a stroke? If so, hypertension was probably the cause. How about heart attacks? Again, hypertension may have been involved. By getting this kind of general information, a pattern often emerges. If this pattern strongly suggests that many members of your family may have had or now suffer from hypertension, you are at increased risk. If you are black, the pattern does not have to be a strong one. Because of the high prevalence of hypertension among American blacks, having one or two family members with high blood pressure is enough to consider yourself at increased risk.

If possible, your detective work should go even further. If your parents or grandparents are living, what are their blood pressures now? Has anyone's pressure risen over the last several years? Even if it has only slightly increased from what it was ten years ago, this should alert you. If it is twenty points higher in systolic pressure or 10 points higher in diastolic pressure—even if these values are still considered "normal" for their age—you are at increased risk.

Fourth—what type of diet do you consume now? Are you a "saltaholic"? Do you automatically add salt when cooking? Do you use the salt shaker immediately before eating a meal? If this is your pattern, you are at increased risk even if none of the other risk factors are present.

Fifth—do you live under excessive tension either at home or at work? Stress is known to raise blood pressure. In fact, the normal response to stress or fear or alarm in all animals is accompanied by a rapid rise in blood pressure. However, when stress is constant, the blood pressure may slowly rise and stay elevated.

The major risk factors for developing hypertension then can be listed as follows:

A blood pressure that is creeping up

Overweight

A family history of hypertension or a tendency to high
  blood pressure

A heavy salt habit in diet

A Type A personality and excessive tension at home or at
  work

By assigning a point value to each of these risk factors
you can calculate your "hypertension score." If your blood
pressure is between 130 and 140 systolic and between 85
and 90 diastolic, score 5. If you are 10 percent above ideal
weight, score 3; 20 percent or more, score 5. If you have
a strong family history of hypertension, score 5; sporadic
family history, score 3. If you are black, add three points.
If you have a Type A personality, score 5; if you are un-
sure, score 1 to 4, depending on the likelihood (similar
to the way you scored for atherosclerosis). Finally, if you
are an obvious saltaholic, score 3. The chart below shows
your hypertension score and should be filled in.

Risk Factor	Maximum Score	Your Score
Blood pressure $\frac{130-140}{85-90}$	5	
Obesity	5	
Positive family history	5	
Black race	3	
Type A personality	5	
Very high salt intake	3	
Total	26	

If your score is below 5, then you are probably not susceptible to hypertension. However, you must remain alert
to the possibility. Stay thin, continue using moderate
amounts of salt, and check your blood pressure regularly.
If your score is 5 or above, you should initiate preventive

measures. These measures involve changing your diet to reduce either your calories or your salt intake, or both.

A Diet for Preventing High Blood Pressure

If you are at high risk for developing hypertension, you will want to reduce your sodium intake. Since salt is by far the most abundant dietary source of sodium, you must begin by reducing your salt intake. Keep the following principles in mind:

Don't add salt at the table.

Don't use extra salt in cooking.

Don't eat smoked or pickled foods.

Use processed foods with the least added salt.

Avoid foods that are naturally high in salt.

You may not be able to accomplish these changes all at once. Many people acquire their taste for salt over many years. It may take months to "unlearn" this habit, but if you are at risk for hypertension it is desirable that you begin breaking the habit as soon as possible.

How Much Salt Reduction Is Enough?

There are three levels of salt reduction: mild, moderate, and strict. Table 6 outlines the steps that need be taken on each of these diets.

Strict sodium restriction is mainly for people who already have hypertension or some other medical condition requiring a very low-sodium diet. However, I believe that there are others who should attempt to reach this kind of control. These are people with a hypertension score of 20 or more who, in addition, are at further risk of developing atherosclerosis because they smoke or have high levels of serum lipids. Although there is no definitive evidence that such people need to reduce their salt intake to such low levels, enough clinical experience has been gathered to suggest that strict control of dietary sodium intake may be beneficial. If you fall into this category it is worth a try. Even if you don't adhere to the strict diet completely, the closer you come the better.

For most people with a score of 5 or more, moderate salt restriction is advisable. While this will definitely require a change in eating habits, this change is not as dif-

TABLE 6   Foods to Omit on a Sodium-Restricted Diet*

Food	*Level of Restriction*		
	Mild	Moderate	Strict
Fruits	*All forms are permitted (including fresh, frozen, canned, and dried)*		
Vegetables, soups, and vegetable juices	*Omit pickled and dehydrated forms*		
		Limit canned to 2 servings daily	Omit all canned and frozen if processed with salt Omit all in Column 2
Meats Fish Poultry Eggs	*Omit cold cuts, sausages, cured and pickled products*		
		Limit canned to 2 servings daily	Omit all canned or frozen with salt
Bread and grain products	*Omit salted crackers, pretzels, etc.*		
		Limit ready-to-eat and "quick cooking" cereals, commercial bread, or baked products to 3 servings daily	Omit all products prepared with sodium

TABLE 6   (*Continued*)

Food	Level of Restriction		
	Mild	Moderate	Strict
Milk and dairy products	*Omit all cheeses and cheese spreads*		
		Limit fluid milk and milk products to 3 servings daily	Omit all but low-sodium products
Seasonings	*Omit bouillon, dehydrated soups, and soy sauce*		
	Limit salt to 1 tsp.	Limit salt to ¼ tsp.	Omit all salt, salted butter, or margarine
	Omit catsup, mustard, commercial salad preparations, and seasoning salts		

*Items in italics apply to all three levels of restriction.

ficult as it might seem. Essentially what it entails is omitting dehydrated soups, bouillon, cold cuts, sausages and other pickled or cured products, salted crackers, pretzels, cheese and cheese spreads, soy sauce, and seasonings such as catsup, mustard, commercial salad preparations, and seasoning salts. In addition, you should limit the amount of all canned vegetables, soups, and vegetable juices to two servings a week. The same is true for all canned meats, fish, poultry, and eggs. Also limit the amount of ready-to-eat quick-cooking cereals and commercial bread or baked products to three servings a day. Finally, limit the amount of milk and milk products to three servings per day, and use no more than one-fourth teaspoon of salt per day in seasoning all foods.

A good way to begin your moderate salt restriction is to take careful stock of what you are currently eating. It is often helpful to record everything you eat for a week.

Examine your record carefully. Where does it differ from the desired pattern of moderate salt restriction? Are you adding more than one-fourth teaspoon of salt to your food? If so, begin to cut back even if you have to do it gradually. Are you eating too many canned goods? This is a common source of excessive sodium intake, since many food processors add large amounts of salt to their products. A few years ago your only alternative was to avoid eating canned goods by using frozen or fresh produce. Today another alternative is becoming more and more practical—the use of canned products that contain no added salt. Read the label! When given a choice of two brands of vegetables, choose the one without added salt. Manufacturers are becoming more aware of the high salt content of our food supply and are finding out that it is good business to have available a low-salt alternative. Even such traditionally salty items as peanuts, potato chips, and pretzels are available now without added salt. By taking a little time and choosing wisely, you can maintain a diet close to what it was before and gain considerable protection against high blood pressure too.

Besides the precautions noted above it is useful to know which foods are naturally high or low in sodium. Table 7 lists vegetables that are high in sodium, and Table 8 lists foods low in sodium permitted at any level of restriction. When it makes no difference to you which vegetable or other food you want, remember these tables and make your choice, keeping the amount of sodium in mind.

TABLE 7   Vegetables Naturally High in Sodium

Artichokes	Celery flakes	Kale
Beet greens	Chard	Mustard greens
Carrots	Dandelion greens	Parsley flakes
Celery		Spinach
		whole hominy
		White turnip

TABLE 8   Foods with Insignificant Amounts of Sodium

Grains	Wheat, oats, rye, rice, barley, and their products (e.g. pasta, breads, flours, uncooked cereals)
Vegetables	All those not in Table 7 or canned/frozen salt-free
Fruits	All fresh/canned fruits and juices
Meats	All fresh or frozen/canned without salt—beef, lamb, pork, veal, poultry, fish, shellfish, and game meats
Eggs	All fresh
Fats	All vegetable oils and shortenings, lard, and unsalted butter and margarine
Condiments	Vinegar, all spices, mustard powder, flavorings (without added salt)
Sweeteners	Sugar, honey, syrup, jellies, molasses
Beverages	Alcoholic beverages, coffee, teas, soft drinks

Planning a Moderate Salt-Restricted Diet

In general, for an adult a diet balanced in the essential nutrients includes at least the following daily servings:

Dairy foods (milk, yogurt, unsalted cheese)	2
Protein foods (meats, poultry, fish, eggs, beans)	2
Fruits	4
Vegetables	3
Breads, cereals, pastas, and rice	4

The following meal suggestions apply to a moderate sodium restriction. When these meals are prepared at home, limit salt to one-fourth teaspoon per day and select the appropriate foods as indicated in Tables 6, 7, and 8.

Breakfast

juice or grapefruit
egg or unsalted cottage cheese
toast

unsalted butter or margarine
cooked cereal (prepared without salt)
milk (whole or skim)
tea or coffee

A Brown-Bag Lunch

sliced chicken, lettuce, tomato, alfalfa sprouts on whole wheat
bread
raisins and nuts (unsalted)
apple
canned fruit juice, coffee, tea, or milk

A Coffee Shop/Short-Order Lunch

hamburger on bun with lettuce and tomato
tossed salad
vinegar and/or oil (not salad dressing)
soda or flavored milk
fruit gelatin

A Dieter's Lunch

unsalted wafers or sandwich bread
hearty tossed salad (with everything except diced cheese and
assorted canned vegetables such as those served at salad
bars) with vinegar and/or oil (as above)
melon half with unsalted cottage cheese
fruit juice, coffee, tea, skim milk (limit use of sodium-based ar-
tificial sweeteners to 2 packets per day)

Evening Meal

broiled codfish
broccoli with lemon sauce
saffron rice (homemade without salt)
dinner roll

unsalted butter or margarine

tossed salad

fruit compote

coffee, tea, or milk

Enhance the variety of your menu at home by making your own mayonnaise and salad dressing. When entertaining, dazzle your guests with some of these tempting items:

Dips

using yogurt as a base, stir in curry powder or black pepper, dill and black pepper, onion and garlic powder (not garlic salt)

Dippers

cherry tomatoes

cold diced cooked white potatoes

fresh beansprouts

sliced green peppers, raw string beans, sliced carrots, sliced celery, etc.

wafers, unsalted crackers, bite-sized sandwich bread, pita bread

Gourmet favorites, such as stuffed mushrooms, pastry puffs, escargots (snails), steamed seafood, meat balls, and aspics can still be served but should be prepared without salt. Experiment with such spices as coriander, cumin, fennel, ginger, and others you never dared try before. When serving dinner for a fancy occasion, convert your favorite recipes to salt-free versions. Vegetables tend not to taste "flat" when they are prepared without salt, and therefore should be incorporated into menus.

When dining out, try to patronize restaurants that cook to order and prepare fresh vegetables. This way you will have more control over the amount of sodium in your food. Oriental restaurants use soy sauce, monosodium glutamate, and other pickled items; as a result, the meals are inescapably high in sodium. Seafood and steak houses may be good choices *if* you can ensure that salt is not added during the preparation of your order. Salads and baked potatoes, which usually accompany entrées, are fairly safe if you forgo dressings and sauces. Fast-food chains and other establishments that serve deep-fried foods have a lot of added salt in their products; here again, a boiled or broiled version of the same food is a better choice.

Your best rule of thumb for a sodium-restricted diet is to follow—literally—the old adage "Take it with a grain of salt."

A mild sodium-restricted diet simply omits pickled and dehydrated vegetables, cold cuts, sausages, and cured or pickled meat and fish products; salted crackers, pretzels, and other snacks; cheese and cheese spreads; bouillon, dehydrated soups, and soy sauce, and it limits any additional salt to 1 teaspoon. Such a regimen is indicated if you have only one risk factor (with the exception of a slowly climbing blood pressure). Thus, anyone with a strong family history of hypertension, or having relatives whose blood pressures have risen with age, or who is obese should use this diet. In addition, if you have independent risk factors for atherosclerosis, such as high serum lipids, or if you are a cigarette smoker, you should use this diet even if your hypertension score is below 5.

For those with scores below 5 and no risk factors for atherosclerosis, the American diet is probably still too high in salt. Although there is no real evidence that any dietary change is necessary for this group, if you are an excessive salt user, you cook with a lot of salt, and salt your food before tasting it, it might be prudent to use the salt shaker more sparingly. Since we do not know all the causes of high blood pressure, you may be prone to this disease even in the absence of all the *known* risk factors. A high salt intake can only aggravate your risk.

Although modifying your diet is extremely important if

your overall hypertension score is too high, you should also direct your attention directly to other life practices that may be contributing to your high score. A Type A personality complicated by environmental stress is very important in this regard. If you have such a personality and live in such an environment—try to modify your behavior. Rest during the day, meditate, exercise, all are valuable tension relievers. Many people relax in different ways; find the way that works for you and that can be applied regularly. This is particularly true if you have any of the other risk factors for high blood pressure. Watching your diet while continuing to live in a pressure cooker isn't enough. Remember high blood pressure has been called the silent killer—you don't know when you have it and if it is not controlled, it can kill with little warning. You owe it to yourself and your family to take all the necessary steps to prevent this disease. Nobody else can do it for you.

Chapter 4

Obesity

There are two primary reasons why obesity is a major health problem in the United States and much of the western world. First, it increases a person's risk for certain of the most serious diseases that afflict our society and second, it can directly impair the quality of our lives even in the absence of one of these diseases. Obesity, therefore, is dangerous because of what it does and because of what it leads to.

In this chapter, I will discuss prevention and treatment of obesity because proper diet is a cornerstone of both. However, before we can have a meaningful discussion of either prevention or treatment, it is very important that we understand what obesity is, how it develops in most people, and why it is dangerous.

The Nature of Obesity

Obesity is not simply being overweight. An obese individual is a person whose body contains too much of one kind of tissue—fat or adipose tissue. The 280-pound linebacker for the New York Jets is not obese, nor is the gold medalist in the women's Olympic shot-put competition, nor is the well-trained heavyweight boxer. These people may be overweight, but almost all their excess weight is in the form of muscle tissue. For most of us, however, over-weight means too much fat tissue, since the body stores excess energy in the form of fat. Therefore, the simplest way of judging whether you have an excess of fat tissue in your body is to examine your weight relative to height. Are you too heavy for your height and body build? Table 9, adapted from the latest Metropolitan Life Insurance Company table, shows the ideal body weights for both men and women of a given height and body build. This table has been constructed from actuarial data and is based mainly on longevity. These are the weights at which people can expect to live longest. Obviously we are talking about population groups, not single individuals, and therefore, although we cannot say that these are necessarily the best figures for you personally, they serve as a good general guide.

As the weight of any population begins to exceed ideal weight the life-span of that population begins to decrease. Look at the table. If you weigh 10 percent above your ideal weight, you are bordering on obesity; a figure of 20 percent above your ideal weight means definite obesity. If your weight is in between, you are in the danger zone. If you are obese, you are at risk of shortening your life-span.

If in your case you are not sure that overweight means too much fat, there are more sophisticated ways of determining the actual amount of fat in your body. Some of these methods, such as the use of skin calipers to measure the thickness of the fat layer on your arms or back, may be used by your physician. The skin-caliper method is useful in differentiating the extremely muscular individual from the person who is equally overweight because of too much fat tissue. This method is also valuable in following the course of weight gain in infants and children, since it may pick up small deviations from the normal pattern which may be an early warning signal for impending obesity. Remember, however, for most of us special techniques like

TABLE 9   1983 Metropolitan Height & Weight Table

	Height			
		Women		
		Small	*Medium*	*Large*
Feet	*Inches*	*Frame*	*Frame*	*Frame*
4	10	102–111	109–121	118–131
4	11	103–113	111–123	120–134
5	0	104–115	113–126	122–137
5	1	106–118	115–129	125–140
5	2	108–121	118–132	128–143
5	3	111–124	121–135	131–147
5	4	114–127	124–138	134–151
5	5	117–130	127–141	137–155
5	6	120–133	130–144	140–159
5	7	123–136	133–147	143–163
5	8	126–139	136–150	146–167
5	9	129–142	139–153	149–170
5	10	132–145	142–156	152–173
5	11	135–148	145–159	155–176
6	0	138–151	148–162	158–179

	Height			
		Men		
		Small	*Medium*	*Large*
Feet	*Inches*	*Frame*	*Frame*	*Frame*
5	2	128–134	131–141	138–150
5	3	130–136	133–143	140–153
5	4	132–138	135–145	142–156
5	5	134–140	137–148	144–160
5	6	136–142	139–151	146–164
5	7	138–145	142–154	149–168
5	8	140–148	145–157	152–172
5	9	142–151	148–160	155–176
5	10	144–151	151–163	158–180
5	11	146–157	154–166	161–184
6	0	149–160	157–170	164–188
6	1	152–164	160–174	168–192
6	2	155–158	164–174	172–197
6	3	158–172	167–182	176–202
6	4	162–176	171–187	181–207

these are not necessary; 10 to 20 percent above ideal weight means danger; more than 20 percent means obesity—too much fat in your body.

Although it is true that obesity simply means too much body fat, the nature of that obesity may vary depending on how that fat is actually stored in our bodies. Like any other tissue, fat or adipose tissue is composed of hundreds of millions of cells (adipocytes or fat cells), each of which contains within its walls a droplet of fat. When the body needs to burn more fat, the droplets shrink. By contrast, when the body needs to store more fat, the droplets swell. Some obese individuals have fat cells that are swollen to three or four times their normal size. Thus, one way to become obese is to blow up your existing fat cells in much the same way as someone might blow up a balloon.

There is a second way, however, in which the body can deposit excess amounts of fat, and that is by creating more fat cells, or speaking figuratively, simply using smaller bricks to build the same-sized wall. Thus, if you are obese your body will always contain too much fat. This fat, however, may be packaged in different ways. You may have a normal *number* of fat cells, each swollen with an excess of fat and therefore *too large*. You may have *too many* fat cells, each containing a normal amount of fat and hence of *normal size*. Or you may be obese as a result of a combination of *too many* fat cells, each of which is *too large*. Figure 1 depicts the different kinds of obesity based on fat-cell number and fat-cell size.

It is important that we understand the differences between these two types of obesity because the nature of the obesity may in large measure determine the success or failure of treatment. In a series of studies, first carried out at the Rockefeller University in New York and since confirmed in many other universities in the United States and abroad, it has been demonstrated repeatedly that weight reduction is always accompanied by a shrinkage in fat-cell size and never accompanied by a reduction in fat-

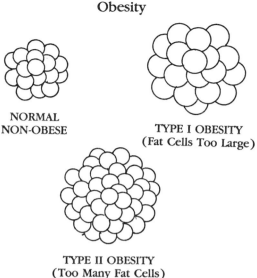

NORMAL
NON-OBESE

TYPE I OBESITY
(Fat Cells Too Large)

TYPE II OBESITY
(Too Many Fat Cells)

hyperplastic and hypertrophic obesity

cell number. If you have too many fat cells, you will always have too many fat cells, no matter how much dieting you do. For example, let us suppose a person has twice as many fat cells as normal and that each cell contains just the right amount of fat. Such a person would be quite obese, since his or her body would contain twice as much total fat as it should. In order for that individual to achieve normal weight, half of the fat from each cell would have to be burned. Thus, the fat cells would shrink to half their normal size. If now we examined the fat tissue of this person, who has painfully dieted down to ideal weight, it would appear more abnormal than when he or she was obese. There would be too many fat cells, which are now too small as well. The body somehow senses this double abnormality and struggles to rectify the situation by trying to fill those "depleted" fat cells with more fat. For this reason it is extremely difficult for a person whose obesity is due primarily to too many fat cells (hyperplastic obesity) to lose weight, and it is even more difficult for that individual to maintain the weight loss for a long time. By

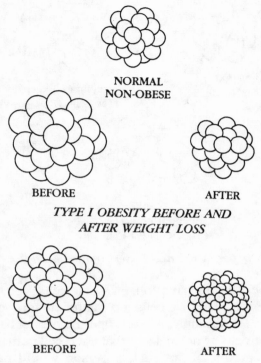

NORMAL
NON-OBESE

BEFORE   AFTER

*TYPE I OBESITY BEFORE AND
AFTER WEIGHT LOSS*

BEFORE   AFTER

*TYPE II OBESITY BEFORE AND
AFTER WEIGHT LOSS*

contrast, let us now examine the obese individual who has
a normal number of fat cells, each containing twice as much
fat as it should. As this person loses weight the fat cells
shrink, and when ideal weight is attained the fat cells are
of normal size. This person's weight is normal, and he or
she has fat tissue composed of a normal number of nor-
mal-sized fat cells. Everything is at the proper level and is
therefore much easier to maintain. Figure 2 depicts how
the adipose tissue might look after weight reduction in
these two types of obesity.

Since the most dangerous form of obesity from the
standpoint of treatability is characterized by an increased
number of fat cells, it is fair to ask how this situation comes

about. Most tissues of the body increase their cell number only during the early phases of their growing period (from fetal life through early childhood). Adipose tissue also adds new cells early in life, although the period during which this can occur extends from before birth to the end of adolescence. Thus, the person who first becomes obese as an adult will simply enlarge the size of already existing fat cells. By contrast, obesity beginning any time during childhood is characterized by an increased number of fat cells. This is why childhood obesity is particularly serious. Although in itself childhood obesity is probably not very dangerous—since children do not suffer from the diseases that occur in obese adults—it almost invariably leads to adult obesity, which is usually the kind that is very difficult to treat. The causes of childhood obesity are very similar to those of adult obesity; the consequences, however, may be quite different.

Fat will be deposited when the energy consumed by your body from the food you eat is greater than the energy expended to keep your body functioning at rest and during exercise. For those of you who are mathematically inclined: energy in = energy out + fat. It seems simple enough; the person who is fat consumes more energy than he expends. For years, however, people have interpreted this to mean that the obese person consumes more food or exercises less than the lean person. Although this may be true for a few obese people, for the vast majority it is not. They simply do not eat more than lean people, and while in general they may exercise less, many will have similar exercise patterns to those of their lean counterparts but still gain weight or remain obese.

Some recent experiments have demonstrated this apparent paradox very dramatically. Obese volunteers spent several weeks in specially constructed rooms in which the amount of energy expended by all forms of exercise could be measured. One obese female patient, when given the same number of calories necessary for a lean woman to maintain her weight, gained weight even though she burned the same number of calories by physical exercise. In order to lose weight she needed to lower her caloric intake to levels below those necessary for the leaner woman to lose weight. Even more impressive was that a person weighing 250 pounds, but whose ideal weight was 150 pounds, first reduced to that weight and then was placed in the type of room described above. In an adjoining room was a woman who was always at her ideal weight of 150 pounds. Both women were fed the same number of calories daily. Both performed the same exercises daily, and measurements showed that both expended the same amount of energy doing the exercises. Yet over the course of several weeks the formerly obese woman gained significant weight, whereas the woman who had been lean all her life remained at the same weight.

The reason for these different responses by obese and lean people is just now beginning to be understood. Most of the energy that we take in with our food supply is expended in keeping our complex body machinery running. Energy is used in every heartbeat, in every breath we take, in the contraction of our stomachs, in the functioning of our kidneys. Energy is used to maintain our body temperature at 98.6°F. The amount of energy necessary to maintain all these functions does vary from person to person. Some people are much more efficient at doing it than others. When food is scarce, the people who utilize energy most efficiently have an advantage. Their bodies run smoothly on fewer calories. They will survive periods of famine longer than their less efficient neighbors. Thus, as the human race evolved in a world constantly plagued by food shortages, the more efficient calorie converters were favored by the process of natural selection. In the last century, however, food has become very abundant in certain countries. Now the efficient calorie converter is no longer at an advantage. In fact, he or she is at a disadvantage. At any given level of intake the individual requires fewer calories to run his metabolic processes, and therefore develops more rapidly a calorie surplus that his body promptly converts to fat.

Thus, the obese individual is a person who handles calories more efficiently; the lean individual, who can eat seemingly endless amounts of calories and not gain weight, is "wasting" calories in maintaining his metabolism. In our food-abundant society this is one situation where inefficiency is definitely rewarded, and obesity is not a punishment for gluttony but a "reward" for efficiency.

Theoretically, then, there are three ways in which an obese individual can lose weight. Reduce the number of calories to such an extent that even an efficient metabolism is left with a deficit. Change the metabolic rate so that it becomes less efficient. Or increase the amount of physical exercise expended so as to burn off the excess fat. In practice, only the first and last alternatives are currently available. There are no good methods for making your body waste calories or change your metabolic rate. Certain drugs can do this either temporarily or permanently, but they are all dangerous. Various diets have been proposed as being able to do so, but all the evidence demonstrates that they do not. And many of these diets can also be dangerous. Thus, until we devise a safe method for altering an obese person's metabolism, the only way to lose weight is to consume fewer calories, exercise more, or both. In this chapter we will discuss the best ways of accomplishing this. However, clearly neither of these options is easy for obese people. Some will have to consume fewer than 1,500 calories per day to keep from gaining weight even if they exercise quite vigorously every day. This is no easy task, to say the least. It is not surprising that most reducing diets fail in the long run to achieve and maintain ideal weight.

The Causes of Obesity

Like most nutritionally related diseases, obesity has several causes. There is a genetic component, which we are just beginning to understand, and a component that is related to life-style. Often the person with a genetic predisposition to obesity becomes obese because of his or her way of life.

Genetics

It has been known for many years that obesity runs in families. If one parent is obese the chances of a child's being obese are about 30 percent. If both parents are obese the chances increase to over 60 percent. These figures alone, however, do not prove that obesity is in any way a genetic disease. Obese parents may simply tend to overfeed their children. In fact, in an attempt to "disprove" the genetic theory of obesity, a study was published several years ago which claimed not only that obese parents had obese children, but that if such a family had a dog, it, too, would likely be obese.

In recent years some studies have demonstrated more directly the importance of genetics in obesity. For example, identical twins raised in different foster homes have tended to conform to the same body type regardless of whether the foster parents were obese. Thus, if one twin was fat the other was fat; if one was lean the other also was lean. These data suggest that the genetic similarity between identical twins was so close that it overrode all the contributions of the children's different environments. By contrast, as the genetic similarity became less close (fraternal twins or siblings), the effect of environment was more noticeable. The children began to assume the body type of the rest of the family in which they were raised. From all these studies we can deduce that two factors definitely contribute to the high incidence of obesity in the children of obese parents; one is the child's genetic background, the other is the environment in which the child is raised.

Recent studies in animals suggest the nature of one type of genetic abnormality in obesity. There are several strains of laboratory rats and mice that are genetically obese. In some of these strains the type of obesity resembles that seen in humans. Early in life the animals lay down too many fat cells. Later in life the fat cells swell to an abnormally large size. Careful studies have shown that beginning at about two weeks of age, the animals' rate of replication of fat cells is faster than normal. Thus, the animals lay down more fat cells because these cells are replicating themselves too quickly. However, this is not the only reason these animals wind up with an enormous increase in fat cells. In normal rats, fat cells stop dividing by one month of age. In genetically obese animals fat-cell division continues until they are at least six months of age. Thus, the genetic abnormality lies in the speed at which the fat cells divide and in the length of time they continue to divide. If we can draw an analogy to humans, it may mean that fat cells continue to divide in genetically prone individuals beyond their adolescence. How much beyond adolescence is not known yet. From a practical standpoint this has enormous implications for both prevention and treatment. Until recently we believed that if we could prevent obesity from occurring in childhood we would be able to eliminate the kind of obesity in which fat-cell number was increased. We know now that this may not be true in certain genetically prone people. In such people, preventing the creation of too many fat cells may mean taking special precautions in early development through to perhaps even middle adult life.

While this cellular abnormality may be the genetic weakness in some obese individuals, in most the genetic factor is probably quite different. As we have seen, many obese people are more efficient in the way they handle calories. The reason why still remains a mystery. However, these people have inherited this increased efficiency from their parents and it puts them at increased risk for obesity. The more efficient you are, the higher your risk. The number of calories that constitutes an excess varies from person to person. Thus, your risk for obesity depends on how efficient you are and how many calories you consume. Your efficiency, as far as we know, is determined genetically. By contrast, the number of calories you consume are at least in part a function of your life-style, and therefore under your control.

Life-style

If we accept the fact that the amount of fat we gain depends on the number of calories we consume minus the number of calories we expend on metabolic processes and on physical exercise, then the only way we can reduce that fat is to reduce the calories we ingest, increase the amount of exercise we do, or both. The problem is that in order to accomplish this, we must often alter our life-style—sometimes radically.

The number of calories a person consumes depends on the amount and the kinds of food he or she eats. However, the quantity and quality of our diets are influenced by a great number of other factors—appetite, culture, religion, ethnicity, social customs, and many others. Therefore, while it is easy to accept that calorie control is the cornerstone of any program designed to prevent or treat obesity, actually limiting the number of calories we consume may be very difficult to achieve.

Let us begin with appetite. Some people appear to be hungry all the time; others consume tiny amounts of food and almost have to force themselves even to do that. Appetite is controlled by a center in our brains called the hypothalamus, which is divided into two areas, one that stimulates appetite and another that inhibits it. In addition, when one of these areas is turned on, it turns the other off. Thus, there is a control mechanism within our brains which can make us eat more or less. In animals, destroying the appetite-stimulating area of the hypothalamus will cause the animal to starve itself to death in the face of an abundance of food. By contrast, destroying the appetite-inhibiting area causes the animal to eat enormous amounts of food and rapidly become obese. There are rare cases of people with tumors of the hypothalamus that have affected their appetite regulation so that they have become markedly obese, whose obesity is cured when the tumors are removed. Both the appetite-stimulating and appetite-inhibiting areas of the hypothalamus are influenced by a network of nerve connections from many other parts of the brain. These nerves, in turn, can be stimulated by "cues" from outside the body (external cues) or from inside the body (internal cues). In other words, your appetite can be stimulated or inhibited by what you see, what you smell, or what you taste, all external cues. It can also be stimulated by contractions in your gastrointestinal tract or even by the thought of a marvelous meal, both internal cues.

Clearly, if we could control our hypothalamus we would have a powerful weapon for combating obesity. We are, however, only just beginning to understand how this complex area of the brain works, and although there are some very exciting studies going on, we have not progressed to the stage where we can safely alter hypothalamic function in obese people. What is known, is that the function of the hypothalamus and, hence, control of appetite differ in obese and lean people. A dramatic example of this difference was demonstrated in a series of studies carried out at Columbia University. Obese and lean individuals had all their food provided in the form of a liquid. The supply of this liquid was kept in a refrigerator which had a drinking tube protruding through one of its walls. Whenever the person was hungry, he or she went to the drinking tube and drank as much as desired. The amount consumed was registered electronically in another room. After a few days each person reached a rather constant caloric intake. Not surprisingly, the obese subjects did not consume many more calories than the lean subjects did. After a few days at this intake level, the liquid diet was changed so that its caloric content was cut in half while its taste and consistency remained the same. The subjects were not told of the change nor did they know it had occurred when they were questioned after the experiment. Lean individuals almost immediately began to consume almost twice as much of the liquid diet. By contrast, obese individuals continued to consume roughly the same quantity as before. Thus, in a lean subject the number of calories being offered was somehow communicated to the hypothalamus, which by regulating the appetite centers was able to control the amount of food taken in. For an obese individual there seemed to be another kind of control operating. Either the hypothalamus was not being influenced by this type of feeding regimen or the volume of liquid (which had not changed during the experiment) was controlling the food intake.

In order to differentiate between these two possibilities, a second series of studies was undertaken. Lean and obese subjects were given access to unlimited quantities of food in a smorgasbord fashion. Again, both lean and obese subjects reached a relatively constant intake over a few days. In this experiment, however, the obese individuals did tend to take in more food than the lean individuals but not enough to account for the obesity. Then the foods were prepared using a sugar substitute, which reduced their caloric content. Again, the subjects were unaware of the change. The lean subjects, as before, simply increased their food intake to reach the caloric level they had previously been consuming. The obese subjects changed their eating patterns very little. In addition, since there was a great variety of foods available and all the subjects had free choice, diets containing markedly different volumes were consumed by individuals in both groups. There was no relationship between the amount of food consumed and the change or lack of change in appetite that occurred when the caloric content was changed. Thus again the lean individuals were responding to an internal cue sent somehow by the body to the brain in response to the number of calories in the diet. By contrast, the obese subjects were not responding either to the caloric content of the food or to the volume consumed. Experiments such as these have led to the theory that the food intake of obese individuals is regulated more by external cues than by internal cues. Or, simply, lean individuals eat when they are hungry for the most part, whereas obese individuals are more likely to eat out of habit, when they are bored, when they are nervous, when they watch television, and so forth. The eating pattern of an obese individual, then, is much more sensitive to certain life-style components not usually associated with diet. What is not yet clear from this research is which came first, the obesity or the altered response of the hypothalamus. Do obese people respond more to external cues because they are obese? Or do people who respond more to external cues tend to *become* obese?

One external cue that for years people have stated is much more sensitive in obese people is a preference for sweet-tasting foods. Obese individuals were said to have a "sweet tooth," and, in fact, this sweet tooth was in large measure responsible for their obesity. Recent studies have demonstrated that neither of these statements is valid. Obese adults given a series of solutions of increasing sweetness preferred the *less* sweet solutions; their lean counterparts did not. This preference persisted even after weight reduction. In obese adolescents the results were somewhat different. They, too, preferred less sweet solutions, but after weight reduction their preference was the same as in the lean subjects. Thus, obese individuals, if anything, have less of a sweet tooth than lean people do, and even after losing weight, they demonstrate no increased preference for sweet foods.

Other recent data suggest that obese subjects *do show* a preference for fat in their diets and that this preference may persist after weight reduction. Since fat contains more than twice as many calories per gram than either carbohydrate or protein, if this finding continues to be valid, it could be extremely important. It suggests that reducing diets which are low in fat may be particularly difficult for obese people to maintain. Since low fat is a cornerstone of most sensible reducing diets, and since Americans consume a relatively high-fat diet, which increases their risk of certain serious diseases, the challenge may be how to reduce the fat in an obese person's diet without destroying his or her incentive to continue that diet.

While much of the research I have described is still not complete, I have gone into some detail so that you can understand why certain approaches to prevention and treatment are used and why other approaches have been discarded. One approach that has had perhaps more success than any other in achieving lasting weight reduction has been behavior modification. This method is based on the premise that by altering your behavior you can minimize your exposure to the external cues that stimulate your appetite center.

As important as appetite is, it alone does not control the number of calories we consume. People do not eat simply because they are hungry. They eat and drink for social reasons. In fact, almost no social occasion can be observed without some kind of food or beverage being served, which is often very high in calories. Even more important is the kind of foods consumed at regular meals. This will vary with a person's ethnic background, family customs, and many other factors. Italians eat quite differently from the Japanese. And even after several generations in the United States, many ethnic differences remain. Religious practices, such as keeping kosher or eating no meat, carry with them certain obvious nutritional implications. Often the kind of foods eaten will determine the number of calories consumed. Seventh Day Adventists are almost always on a relatively low-calorie diet. Eastern European Jews often eat more fat and hence have a relatively higher-calorie diet than do Orientals. Therefore, any weight-reduction program must take into account that person's eating habits. There is no use trying a diet that consists of foods you will not be able to incorporate into your way of life. Even if you can stay on such a diet for a short time and you do lose some weight, you will gain it back as soon as you resume your previous eating habits.

Exercise
The amount of physical exercise you perform will affect your weight in two ways. First, exercise burns calories directly. Table 10 shows the number of calories expended during various types of athletic activities.

Second, exercise, in some still not understood manner, causes the body to consume more energy than can be accounted for by the amount of physical work performed. Whether certain exercises cause the body to become less "efficient" in handling calories is still unclear. However, some experts believe that this is an important mechanism by which exercise aids in weight reduction.

To summarize, obesity occurs when the body is taking in more energy than it is expending. This condition can occur in anyone consuming a large enough number of calories. In most obese individuals, however, it occurs at caloric intakes that are not greater than the caloric intakes of lean individuals. The obese person may handle calories more efficiently and hence at the same caloric intake as a lean person, will have an excess, one that is turned into fat! To treat obesity, however, we must reduce the number of calories consumed or increase the amount of physical exercise performed. We must employ one or both

TABLE 10   Calorie Expenditures per Hour for
         Different Activities *

Activity	Calories Expended per Hour of Continuous Exercise
Bicycle riding	200–600
Walking moderately fast	200–300
Football	560
Soccer	560
Frisbee	200
Basketball	500
Tennis	500–700
Volleyball	300
Swimming	300–600
Dancing	200–400
Jogging	400–500
Skiing (cross-country)	650–1,000
(downhill)	350–500

*Based on an individual weighing approximately 130–150 lbs. Add
more calories if the person is heavier.

of these techniques because as yet we are unable to alter
the body's metabolism safely to make it a less efficient
calorie converter.

Thus, the treatment of obesity does not really get at the
core of the problem. In order to reduce caloric intake we
must try to decrease appetite, an appetite which may be
perfectly normal. This is not an easy job. We must try to
alter the pattern of food intake and the kind of foods eaten,
a pattern that may be deeply rooted in religion, ethnicity,
and family background. Again, this is not an easy job. Finally, we can try to increase the amount of exercise. This
approach is an excellent one to use in the prevention of
obesity but of limited use in its treatment. Is it any won-
der that more people are cured of even the most malig-
nant type of cancer than are permanently cured of obesity?
What happens, then, to those people not cured of obes-

ity? Is it worth the effort a person must go through or is our society too concerned with being overweight? Is the billion-dollar-a-year diet industry making any impact on our health? In order to answer these questions, let us examine the health consequences of obesity.

The Consequences of Obesity

1. Obesity increases your chances for developing three of the major risk factors for atherosclerosis: high blood pressure, high blood levels of cholesterol, and diabetes. In addition, obesity increases your risk directly for gall bladder disease and certain forms of cancer. Thus, obesity can result in premature death directly and indirectly.

2. Obesity by itself can result in health liabilities such as shortness of breath, increased risk for any surgical procedure, and a greater propensity for certain kinds of accidents.

3. Obesity will result in major restrictions on a person's living habits and can interfere with the quality of life in general. The obese individual is a member of an oppressed minority, and is often viewed by society not only as deformed but deformed through his or her own gluttony.

If you are obese you should be concerned about these three problems. It is ironic of course that the third problem, which in many ways is the most serious an obese person faces, is not really his or her problem but that of the society in which he or she lives. In Polynesia if you are obese, you are literally worth your weight in gold. In the United States, at best, society pities you. As we shall see, the health risks attributed to being overweight, while real, are minimal for most individuals. If only people who were truly obese and at increased risk for major health problems were to undertake serious weight-reduction schemes, publishers would be in trouble and a billion-dollar diet industry would shrink to nothing. Let us therefore examine obesity as a major health risk.

How Obesity Affects Your Health

At the beginning of this chapter I defined obesity as 20 percent above your ideal weight. In this section I am not discussing the person who is five, ten, fifteen, or even twenty pounds overweight. What I am saying is that if you *should* weigh 150 pounds, you are obese at 180 pounds; and if you *should* weigh 180 pounds, you are obese if you weigh 216 pounds.

There is no evidence that people who are overweight but not obese are at any significantly increased risk for any of the major diseases listed above. Your ideal weight is the weight that offers you the greatest longevity statistically; the curve rises sharply only after you are well into the obesity range. For practical purposes, then, you should begin to worry about overweight potentially shortening your life when you approach the obesity range. For that reason I have indicated that if you are 10 to 20 percent above ideal weight, you may be in a danger zone. If you are in this zone you do not necessarily need to lose weight. What is much more important is that you don't gain any more weight. A person who is 10 percent above ideal weight and has been that way for ten years, may only need to keep careful watch on his or her weight. By contrast, a person whose weight has always been at or close to ideal, but then begins to creep up slowly but steadily and reaches the 10 percent mark, should begin an active program to stop any further weight gain.

Once you have reached the obesity range, your risk for the abnormalities and diseases listed above is increased. But the risk does not increase linearly the heavier you get. At most, there is a small increase in risk until you are moderately to severely obese. The actual number of pounds you can sustain before this sharp increase in risk occurs will vary from person to person and with the abnormality or disease in question. Thus, you may have to be forty pounds overweight before your risk for high blood levels of cholesterol has increased significantly, and perhaps thirty pounds for high blood pressure or diabetes. These figures are just examples. What I am trying to point out is that even if you are technically obese, your risk may not be increased very much if you are at the lower end of the spectrum.

I am not going into all this detail just to make an abstract point. I am also not saying that if you are mildly obese, don't worry about it. What I am saying, however, has very practical value in weight reduction. The most important objective of any weight-reduction program should be to lower your risk for the diseases we have discussed. Therefore, it is much more important that you lose enough weight to change your risk category than it is to reach your "ideal" weight. One major reason most reducing programs fail is that we set inappropriate goals. For the man whose ideal weight is 180 but who weighs 240, a loss of twenty-five pounds may reduce his risk markedly, even though it won't change his physical image very much. What is most important, however, is that a loss of twenty-five pounds may be attainable and sustainable, whereas if he attempts to lose forty or fifty pounds, he will almost surely fail and will wind up not only back where he started, but extremely frustrated and bitter.

As we have seen in Chapters 2 and 3, atherosclerosis and hypertension both involve multiple risk factors. We shall see in Chapter 5 that the same holds true for diabetes. Atherosclerosis, hypertension, and diabetes are the three major killer diseases to which obesity makes a significant contribution (since obesity increases the risk only slightly for just a few, relatively rare cancers). The nature of this contribution is still not entirely clear. Careful analysis of available data has led some experts to believe that in these diseases, obesity is important only if you already have a genetic predisposition to any or all of them and then only if you are severely obese. If you fall into this category, you are at high risk and should make every effort to lower your weight sufficiently to reduce that risk. If you do not fall into this category and are very obese, while there is certainly no room for complacency, weight reduction may be less of an emergency.

I am sure many of you reading this chapter are above your ideal weight. Before considering a crash diet assess your personal condition. Are you obese? If so, how obese? Do you have a positive family history for atherosclerosis, high blood pressure, or diabetes? Are you in the danger zone we discussed above? Only after you have answered these questions honestly can you decide whether weight reduction will improve your health and how much is necessary in your particular case.

Preventing Obesity

Perhaps with no other disease is the old adage "An ounce of prevention is worth a pound of cure" as true as with obesity. It is therefore well worth the trouble to assess your risk for becoming obese and, if you are in danger, to do something about it before it is too late.

As we have seen, there is a strong genetic component to obesity. Therefore, your family history is important; if your family health tree shows obesity, your own tendency to become overweight is increased. Even if there is no history of obesity in your family, a careful examination of the rest of your family history is still important. Since obesity is particularly dangerous when coupled with a genetic propensity for high blood-cholesterol levels, high blood pressure, or diabetes, a history of any of these conditions in your family background makes your being obese more dangerous. In other words, while a positive family history for any or all these abnormalities will not increase your risk for obesity, conversely, if you do become obese, your risk for heart attack or stroke will increase.

If you were obese as a child, you are at increased risk of being obese as an adult, and you must consider yourself at risk even if your weight is normal now.

Beyond your own history and your family history, consider your life-style very carefully. Are you becoming more sedentary because of your age, your job, or just because of a new way of life? Are you a complusive eater whose appetite is triggered by external cues, especially during periods of tension? Have you increased your consumption of alcohol, which is a source of hidden calories? If the answer to any of these questions is yes, you are at increased risk. Finally, if you are a woman and have children, did you gain a little weight permanently after each pregnancy? Do premenstrual tensions result in your eating more? Again, if the answer is yes, your risk is increased.

Scoring Your Personal Risk for Obesity

First, your present weight: if you are 10 to 20 percent above ideal weight, you are in the danger zone, and you should score 5.

Second, your family history—on a scale of 1 to 5: if your family health tree is abundant with obese relatives, score 3; if your father or mother was obese, score 4; if both parents were obese, score 5.

Third, your own history: if you were truly obese as a child, score 5. If you have always had a problem controlling your weight, score 3.

Fourth, your life-style: if you are a compulsive eater, score 2 to 5, depending on how much tension you are under and how much food you consume during periods of tension. If you live a moderately sedentary life, score 2; if you do almost no exercise; score 4. If you are a moderately heavy drinker, add 2; and if you are a woman and have slowly been getting heavier with each pregnancy, add

TABLE 11

Risk Factor	Maximum Score	Your Score
10–20% above ideal weight (danger zone)	5	
History of childhood obesity	5	
Family history of obesity	3–5	
Compulsive eater	2–5	
Sedentary life	2–4	
Moderate alcohol consumption	2	
Increased weight after each pregnancy	2	
Total	21–28	

2. Table 11 lists the risk factors for obesity and their scores.

A score of 5 or more places you at risk for obesity. As your score increases, your risk rises, but anyone scoring 5 or above should take measures to prevent obesity from occurring.

If you actually suffer from atherosclerosis, or have high blood-cholesterol levels or high blood pressure or diabetes, you should institute preventive measures against obesity, even if you are of normal weight. I would also advise instituting preventive measures even if you do not actually suffer from those diseases but do have a strong family history for one or more of them. Again, your risk for obesity may not be increased but the potential danger of becoming obese is greater.

Watching Your Diet

There is no specific number of calories that must be consumed to prevent obesity. What is right for you may be too much for your friend even though you are both of the same age, sex, and body build. You have to find your own level. Begin by checking your weight several times a week. If it is stable and you are not in the danger zone, continue to check it but note the amount of food you take in and estimate your average daily caloric intake.

That is all you have to do except to check your weight once a week. As long as it remains stable, no other measures are necessary. If your weight begins to increase, even by one or two pounds, recalculate your caloric intake. If your intake has gone up, cut back to where it was before. This may be difficult to do if your eating pattern has changed, and it may necessitate modifying your pattern somewhat. We shall see that by instituting some simple measures you may nip a potentially serious problem in the bud.

If you are in the danger zone (10 to 20 percent above ideal weight) and your weight is stable, you need to lose some pounds but you have plenty of time in which to do it. You can decrease the number of calories you consume, increase the amount of physical activity you perform, or both. Don't go on a crash program to drop your weight below the danger zone. You will just bounce back after the program is over. The majority of Americans who are on crash diets at any given time are either in the danger zone or are even less overweight; only a relative few are actually obese. Remember, you are not at increased health risk. You should lose some weight to *prevent* yourself from *becoming* obese later in life when there is a tendency to gain more weight. If you take your time making a few changes in your diet and your life-style and don't try to reach your ideal weight but aim instead for any weight below the danger zone that you can comfortably sustain, you are much more likely to succeed in losing those pounds.

To be sure, you will have to reduce the number of calories you take in. The best way to do this is to identify the sources of calories in your diet that contain the lowest nutrient value. The principle I am trying to convey is not to go on any special diet but rather to modify the one you are on now so as to reduce the number of calories in it without affecting the number of nutrients it contains. Obviously, if your diet has been poorly balanced to start with, it may still be poorly balanced and probably should be changed. The time to change it is after you have reached the proper caloric level and sustained that level for several months, not when you are beginning a program to lose weight. The less radical the change as you begin to limit your calories, the better.

Which foods or elements in your diet are the source of these unwanted calories? This will vary with different people. For some, it may be alcohol; for others, refined sugar; for others, fat; and for many, all three. Which should you cut out? It doesn't really matter as long as you reach the caloric level that will begin to bring about weight reduction.

There are some general rules to help you decide what foods to eliminate or reduce in quantity. Fat has twice the number of calories per gram as sugar. Thus, eliminating a given quantity of fat reduces your calories twice as much as eliminating the same amount of sugar. Suppose you consume 2,500 calories per day from the following foods: whole milk, toast and butter, coffee (three cups a day) with two teaspoons of sugar, tunafish or chicken salad sandwich, steak, home-fried potatoes, vegetable, salad, cheesecake, or apple pie—a pretty standard American diet. In addition, you have one martini before dinner and a glass or two of wine with dinner.

You want to reduce your intake to 2,200 calories. What are your options? First, identify those sources of calories which have little or no nutrient value:

Alcohol—Cutting out the martini will save calories.

Sugar—Eliminating the sugar from your coffee or substituting a noncaloric sweetener saves calories.

Fat—Carefully trimming your meat and having a baked potato (without butter or sour cream) may save calories. Eliminating the butter from your toast, the mayonnaise from your sandwich, or using skim milk may save calories. A simple change from creamy salad dressing to oil and vinegar saves calories.

Combined fat and sugar—Replacing the cheesecake or apple pie with a piece of fruit can reduce your caloric intake by more than 100 calories.

The number of ways in which you can eliminate 300 calories and still keep the nutrient value of your diet essentially the same is almost infinite. And you don't have to do it the same way each day. The most important thing is to be aware of what you are eating and to initiate the kind of changes that are easiest for you.

Modifying Your Behavior

Sometimes the number of calories you consume can begin to creep up because of a change in your life-style. For example, a promotion in your job which makes it necessary to entertain clients at lunch once or twice a week, or a simple change from eating in the company cafeteria to the executive dining room, can increase your caloric intake enough to result in a slow weight gain. Be alert to this possibility, and if you do begin to gain, cut back your calories to the previous number. This doesn't mean you have to give up your new life-style. It means you have to adapt it to the number of calories that help maintain your weight at a healthy level. Maybe ordering differently at lunch is the answer, or perhaps modifying your dinner, or a combination of the two. Choose whatever method works best for you. Once your caloric intake is at its previous level and you have shed the extra pound or two, continue this pattern of eating while continuing to weigh yourself several times a week. In most cases you will have stabilized at your previous weight and will have averted a potentially serious weight problem.

Often changes in life-style occur so subtly that they may go unnoticed for a long time. Sometimes these changes can be accompanied by significant weight gain, perhaps even fifteen or twenty pounds. The gradual shift from the active exercise pattern of high school and college to the less active pattern of a young man or woman entering the workforce can often result in a weight gain. Increasing your alcohol intake, giving up smoking, traveling more often for business or pleasure, all may be accompanied by an increased intake of calories and a slow but steady increase in your weight. If you are at risk for obesity, you should be constantly on the alert for these changes; anticipate them and adjust your calorie intake accordingly. Remember, there is an infallible measure of success which you can read right on your bathroom scale.

Finally, there are certain activities which are usually accompanied by eating. Who can go to the movies without eating some popcorn? A baseball game without a hot dog or soft drink is not complete. Part of going to the theater is the coffee and pastry you have after the show. All these activities enrich our lives and to suggest giving them up is neither necessary nor practical. If they occur occasionally, don't worry. If they form a regular and frequent part of your life, then the calories you consume at these times must be considered as part of your overall calorie allowance. What is important is that you be aware of what you are actually eating and that you change the pattern in a way that preserves the social event and at the same time eliminates unwanted calories.

Perhaps the most important factor directly contributing to obesity is the television set. Watching television is a sedentary activity. In addition, for many it is also a time for unconscious eating. Finally, at least half the commercials are for food or beverages. Analyze your television viewing time. Are you a beer and pretzels football-game watcher? Do you nibble on candy or crackers throughout your favorite programs? For several evenings just write down everything you eat as you watch. Then calculate the calories: how many? 500? 750? Find a way to bring that number down. Put the peanuts on the top shelf of the closet. Substitute fruit for pretzels and juice or sugar-free iced tea for beer. You don't need a prescribed plan to tell you how to reduce your television calories. You just need to be aware that you are consuming calories as you watch; you need to know how many you are consuming; and you need the determination to alter this pattern and reduce your caloric intake. There is no one way to do it. There is no best way to do it. If one method fails try another. Use any method that works for you, but control the amount and kind of food and keep the number of calories to a level that sustains your weight and prevents it from creeping up.

Exercise

Between the ages of twenty-five and fifty, Americans do not increase their food intake to any great extent. Think of yourself. Do you eat more now than when you were twenty-five? If anything, you probably eat less. And yet between the ages of twenty-five and fifty all of us tend to gain weight. This gain is due partly to changes in our metabolism, but mainly it is a result of a steady decline in physical activity. I don't mean sports or other planned exercise. I am talking about physical activity in the normal course of the day's events.

My former college roommate is a pediatrician in Phoenix, Arizona. He is interested in physical fitness and has clocked the amount of walking he does (outside of planned exercise) in one day. It is less than one mile! He drives to work, to stores; he even drives to the exercise activities in which he regularly participates. He asked me to clock my mileage. Using the same pedometer as he used, I registered three miles a day. I live in New York and each day I walk from my home to the bus stop, from the bus stop to my office, and the reverse. Then from my home I walk with my wife to the supermarket, or to a neighborhood restaurant. I average three miles per day. My former roommate and I both do the same kind of sedentary work and yet the nature of the place in which I live causes me to walk 750 miles a year more than he does. In the twenty-five years since we began our professions, in the course of my everyday activities I have walked 18,750 miles more than my colleague has. Yet no one who knows us would say that I am more active. I give you this example because I hope it surprises you as much as it surprised me. It points out differences in activity, which over time can be of enormous magnitude, but which for the most part can go unnoticed. Simply walking several more miles in the course of a day or taking the staircase instead of the elevator can make a big difference. The key, however, is regularity; make exercise part of your regular daily routine. Think about how you can introduce more activity into this routine. In some ways this might be the greatest challenge we all face in our struggle to prevent obesity.

Of course, regular physical activity will increase both your caloric expenditure and your physical fitness if you are relatively sedentary. My former roommate jogs or walks briskly ten miles every day. Some people play tennis, others work out in gyms, but whatever activity it is, to help prevent obesity it should be done on a regular basis. It must become an integral part of your life-style. Therefore, it is essential that you enjoy it. Don't run because everyone else does if running bores you; you'll never sustain it. If you like to dance, do it regularly. Take a daily walk—to the office, the supermarket, a friend's house. Ride a bicycle; swim if you have access to a pool. Any of these activities will consume calories. The best one is not the one that consumes the most calories but the one you can make a part of your daily routine. Whatever you do, remember, your bathroom scale will tell you if you are being successful.

Treatment of Obesity

There are two major incentives that must be kept in mind in treating your obesity:

1. You wish to reduce your body weight to a range that lowers your risk for the complications of obesity.

2. You wish to institute preventive measures against atherosclerosis and high blood pressure, both of which are more common in obese people.

Unfortunately, true obesity is an affliction which more often than not will plague you the rest of your life. Most obese people have tried numerous diet plans, lost and regained hundreds of pounds, and have had little permanent success in controlling their weight. Therefore, while it is important that you try to lose weight, it is equally important that you accept the possibility that you may always be obese and try to protect yourself from its complications.

Reducing Your Body Weight

This is not a diet book. I have no intention of prescribing the "perfect diet" which in three weeks will take off thirty pounds. No such diet exists! For an obese person to lose significant weight and to keep it off means a lifetime of hard work. However, I am going to give you some tips that might help lessen the burden of constantly watching your diet. Remember, you may not be an overeater; instead, you may be an underuser of calories. This means that you may have to reduce your number of calories to a level below that which a nonobese individual would have to consume for you to lose weight. The number of calories you can take in while still losing weight will vary from person to person. For some obese individuals, 2,000 per day will achieve weight loss; for others, 1,500; for some, 1,200 or even less. Find your level and construct your own diet by eliminating fat and sugar and alcohol, and by using foods whose caloric value totals the necessary number of calories per day. If you find that you must consume 1,500 calories or less to begin a slow but steady weight loss, take a multivitamin and mineral supplement. Any brand that gives you the recommended daily allowances of B vitamins, vitamin C, iron, zinc, and calcium is right. Do not use megavitamin pills; they are unnecessary and can be dangerous.

Continue at this caloric level until you stop losing weight. This will often occur after two to three weeks. What is happening is that your initial weight loss is partly water and the resulting tissue dehydration is correcting itself. You are still losing fat tissue, but the scale isn't showing it because you are ·replacing water at the same time. Be patient! In another week, after you are rehydrated you will begin to lose weight again. After another few weeks, you may reach another plateau. Your metabolism is fighting you and increasing its efficiency. This is not the time to give up but rather the time to fight back. Reduce your caloric intake by 100 to 200 calories. Your weight will begin to decrease again.

The procedure I have outlined does not take two weeks or two months. It takes much longer: six months, nine months, twelve months, depending on how obese you are and also on your metabolism.

Remember, your goal is not to achieve ideal weight but one that will minimize the risks of obesity. Any weight that is below the danger zone is excellent. Even if this results in your being within the danger zone, you are much better off than you were before. Here is an example. Suppose you weigh 250 pounds and your ideal weight is 180 pounds; 110 percent of your ideal weight would be 198 pounds, so at 216 pounds you are obese. Thus, to reach ideal weight you must lose seventy pounds and maintain that weight loss; to be below the danger zone you have to lose fifty-two pounds and maintain that weight. To be no longer obese you will have to lose thirty-four pounds and maintain that weight. Thus, you need to lose half as much weight to be no longer obese than to achieve your ideal weight. However, by losing those thirty-four pounds you reduce your risk of the complications of obesity perhaps by *80 percent or more*. The next thirty-six pounds will only reduce your risk by an additional 15 to 20 percent. Certainly, you would be best off to achieve and maintain your ideal weight, but experience has taught us that this goal is almost unattainable. Therefore, you are advised to set a goal you can attain and which at the same time eliminates the major portion of your risk.

Maintain that weight until it becomes your new stable weight. Then if you wish to take off more weight, that's fine. If you succeed you will have reduced your risk a little bit more and have obtained important cosmetic and psychological effects. If you fail and return to your new baseline, you will still be at much lower risk than when you started.

Keeping your weight stable with the least amount of caloric restriction possible is easier the more active you are. Therefore, when you reach your desired goal, begin a moderate exercise routine which can be incorporated into your new low-calorie eating habits. Exercise will not only help you keep your new weight, but may *directly* reduce your risk for atherosclerosis and hypertension and their most dreaded complication—heart attack.

Recommendation for Reducing Your Risk

I wish I could have ended this chapter at the end of the last section. Obviously the best way to minimize the risks of obesity is to lose sufficient weight so you *are* no longer obese. Unfortunately, even if they set proper goals, many obese individuals will not or cannot permanently reduce their weight. These people are at increased risk for a number of diseases, two of which—high blood pressure and atherosclerosis—can be influenced by diet. If you are obese and have not been able to reduce your weight, you should be constantly alert for these diseases. Your blood pressure should be taken at least twice a year and your serum lipids should be analyzed with the same frequency. If you have a serum cholesterol above 200, you should alter your diet as set forth in Chapter 2. If you are a male with a family history of atherosclerosis and you are obese, you should institute this low-fat diet even if you have no other risks for atherosclerosis. If you are a female with marked obesity (30 percent or more above ideal weight) with a positive family history for atherosclerosis you should similarly modify your diet.

As for hypertension, obesity itself is reason enough to reduce the amount of salt in your diet (see Chapter 3). If you are black or have a family history of high blood pressure, you must be even more careful of your salt intake. Beyond these dietary changes, it is important to have your blood pressure carefully monitored, as it may go up even if you modify your salt intake. Today, very effective drug therapy exists for hypertension (high blood pressure). The key is to begin early and this can be done only if you are aware that your blood pressure is high. If you are obese you are more at risk for hypertension, and therefore must take special pains to start controlling this disease, if it does occur, as early as possible. Your life may depend on it.

Chapter 5

Diabetes

Diabetes, with its dreaded complications, is one of the most serious and common chronic diseases in modern society. Diabetes results from a deficiency of insulin, a hormone produced by the pancreas, an organ that lies buried in the abdomen behind the liver and intestines.

Diabetes, however, can be viewed as two separate diseases. One form, usually affecting younger people—even young children—is due to an *absolute* deficiency of insulin. The mechanism within the pancreas that normally manufactures insulin becomes badly damaged and can no longer produce the hormone. This type of diabetes, often called juvenile-onset diabetes, is very severe and must be treated promptly with insulin, which the patient must take for the rest of his or her life. Juvenile-onset diabetes is quite rare, and while diet is a mainstay in its treatment, as we shall see there is no way to prevent its occurrence through dietary modification.

The second form of diabetes is often called maturity-onset or adult-onset diabetes. It also results from a deficiency of insulin, but this deficiency is a *relative* one. The pancreas is perfectly capable of manufacturing the hormone; in fact, it often manufactures more than it did before. What happens is that the body needs more hormone to function properly. Certain changes have taken place within the tissues which increase their requirement for insulin. The pancreas responds by making more. First it works at increased capacity and finally it works at maximum capacity. If the requirement continues to increase, the pancreas simply cannot manufacture enough insulin. The patient becomes insulin-deficient and the symptoms of diabetes appear. Sometimes if the situation is not relieved, the overworked pancreas will "burn itself out," thus becoming unable to manufacture insulin efficiently. What started out as a *relative* deficiency can then become an *absolute* deficiency. This second type of diabetes is much more common than the first, and we shall see that in certain people the risk of acquiring the disease may be lowered by dietary modification.

In this chapter I shall discuss dietary modifications that can lower the risk for adult-onset diabetes in high-risk people as well as principles in the dietary management of diabetes when the disease is already present. Remember that anyone with either type of diabetes must be under a doctor's care. The dietary principles that I will outline will make it easier to understand why your doctor is prescribing a particular type of diet. If there seems to be a difference between what is outlined below and what your doctor is prescribing, discuss it with him or her. In the last analysis, however, your physician knows your particular case, and, hence, as long as you are under his or her care, you should follow his or her dietary instructions.

Juvenile-Onset Diabetes

Juvenile-onset diabetes is a disease with a very definite genetic component. In fact, the actual genes involved have been located so that it is possible to predict (after certain specialized tests have been done) which individual is at risk for this disease. However, trying to make this prediction currently offers little advantage to the person who is at risk. Only a small number of this population will actually develop diabetes, and nothing can be done either to identify or to protect this group. At present, we believe that some people with this genetic predisposition are either more sensitive to a common virus or more susceptible to an uncommon virus. Whichever the case, the cells within the pancreas that produce insulin are selectively destroyed by what appears to be a viral infection. The person rapidly becomes ill and dies within a matter of months unless diagnosed and treated promptly. Before the availability of insulin, all patients with true juvenile-onset diabetes died within a short time. Today, with the availability of insulin, most can live a relatively normal life. However, such patients become susceptible to the same long-term complications of diabetes as those who develop the adult form of the disease. Since the dietary modifications designed to lower a person's risk for these complications are similar for both types of diabetes they will both be discussed. However, as far as dietary controls to prevent juvenile diabetes are concerned, there are none. There is no relationship to the number of calories consumed, the amount of carbohydrate, either complex or simple, the amount of refined sugar or fat in the diet. Don't listen to nutritional "experts" who tell you you got diabetes because you were too fat (most juvenile-onset diabetics are thin) or that you ate too much candy, or ice cream, or sugar. And above all, don't feel guilty. Nothing you did or did not do caused your diabetes.

Maturity-Onset Diabetes

This is a type of diabetes which typically begins after the age of fifty, which runs in families, and for which we will develop a risk profile because dietary modification may be able to lower that risk. To do this, however, we must understand how this relative insulin deficiency develops, since it is this pattern of development that we will attempt to alter by dietary modifications.

The Action of Insulin

The hormone insulin is produced by special cells (beta cells) which are present in small clumps or islands interspersed between the ducts of the pancreas. These islands, called islets of Langerhans (after the man who discovered them), have a characteristic appearance under the microscope. The insulin manufactured in the beta cells is secreted directly into the bloodstream and is carried to all the tissues of the body. The cells of these tissues have specific molecular appendagelike protrusions from their surface into which the insulin molecules fit and are thereby bound to the cell surface. These appendages are called receptors and they are specific for insulin. Usually there are more receptors than insulin to fill them. Thus, as the demand goes up, more insulin is produced, immediately becomes fixed to a receptor, and is rapidly taken into the cell. If for some reason some or all of the receptors are not working properly, the pancreas will have to produce more insulin for the same amount actually to get into the cells. There is some evidence suggesting that obesity alters the receptors on the fat cells to make them less efficient.

Once inside the cell, insulin facilitates the passage of glucose, the body's main energy source, from the blood into the tissues, which will either use it as fuel or store it as fat or as the complex carbohydrate glycogen. In the case of the fat cells, insulin opens the door for glucose to enter and be converted to fat. When excess calories are consumed, the body stores them as fat. In order to do this, more insulin is required than when caloric intake is lower. Thus, in order to build up or maintain fat stores, an obese individual requires more insulin than a lean individual. The beta cells are forced to work harder as the body's need for insulin increases. If they can meet that need, the body will function normally. If they cannot, there is a *relative* insulin deficiency and the symptoms of diabetes will appear. In some people the added need for insulin is no problem for the beta cells. They simply make more and pump it out into the bloodstream. In others the cells cannot make it fast enough. Which type of person you are depends on your genetic makeup. Maturity-onset diabetes is a genetic disease that manifests itself when the body's requirement for insulin increases. Under normal circumstances a person who is at risk for the disease because he or she is carrying "diabetic genes" may actually develop it at age sixty-five or seventy, or even older. However, if an added strain is put on the pancreatic beta cells, diabetic symptoms may appear when that person is in the fifties or even younger. People who are prone genetically to the disease will develop it much sooner and much more seriously if they consume large amounts of calories. Calories, however, can come from a variety of sources, and some people have claimed that some of these sources are more dangerous than others.

The actual signal that stimulates the pancreatic beta cells to make more or less insulin is the level of blood glucose. As the level increases, more insulin is made. As it decreases, less is made. Insulin is needed to get the glucose into the cells. As this occurs, the amount of glucose in the blood will fall. Thus, another function of insulin is to regulate the level of blood sugar. The level of blood sugar is also sensitive to dietary factors, particularly to the amount of carbohydrate in the diet. Complex carbohydrates must first be converted to simple forms in the intestine before they are absorbed into the body. Thus, they release sugar into the blood slowly. Refined sugar (sucrose) is split into its two simple sugars, glucose and fructose, very quickly by the intestines and these are absorbed into the bloodstream extremely rapidly. Hence, consumption of sucrose will raise blood sugar more rapidly than the consumption of complex carbohydrate.

Many people have postulated that a diet high in refined sugar will put an added strain on the beta cells and that over a long time, such a diet will induce diabetes in susceptible individuals. Several studies have been cited in an attempt to reinforce this hypothesis. Unfortunately, none of these studies was controlled in the scientific sense of a controlled study. Thus, there may be an association between high intake of refined sugar with diabetes because people who consume large amounts of sugar also consume large numbers of calories. And we have already seen that too many calories can increase a susceptible individual's risk for diabetes. Certainly to the extent that consuming large amounts of sucrose increases your caloric intake, it is a risk factor for maturity-onset diabetes. However, there is nothing special about sugar beyond its caloric content that increases the risk for diabetes.

This point is of more than academic interest when it comes to designing a diet that will help protect a person at high risk. To lower calories in our society the best way is to reduce your intake of fat. This is particularly important in a person who has diabetes as well as in someone who is at high risk for developing the disease. A low-fat diet will necessarily be high in carbohydrate. A low-carbohydrate diet is relatively high in fat. Therefore, it is very difficult to construct a diet low in both these components. If both the number of calories and the amount of carbohydrate increased your risk for diabetes independently, both dietary prevention and treatment would be very complicated. Luckily this is not so. Calories are important; however, the amount of complex carbohydrate consumed is not. In fact, there is evidence that a diet high in complex carbohydrate may be particularly beneficial in treating diabetes. As far as refined sugar is concerned, the jury is still out. Certainly very large amounts must be avoided because such a diet will provide a low-bulk, pleasant source of calories. However, if calories are controlled, severe restriction of refined sugar is probably not necessary as a preventive measure for maturity-onset diabetes.

Who Is at Risk?

Anyone with a family history of diabetes is at risk for developing the disease. The stronger the family history, the greater the risk. The closer the relationship, the greater the risk. Another important factor in determining the importance of the genetic component of your risk is the time diabetes actually appeared in those members of your family tree who developed it. The earlier the onset of the disease, the more you are at risk. Since life expectancy has increased dramatically in recent years, and since diabetes may appear late in life, even a family tree totally devoid of diabetes is not absolute assurance of a lack of genetic risk.

If you belong to a group in which the risk for diabetes is high, you also are at least potentially at risk. Among these high-risk groups are Ashkenazi Jews, blacks, and Amerindians. If you belong to one of these groups, you should examine your family tree very carefully. If information about certain close relatives is unavailable, you may have to consider yourself at increased risk. Since the dietary modifications to reduce this risk are simple, safe, and useful in protecting against other diseases (atherosclerosis, hypertension, and obesity), it is better to err on the safe side in deciding your risk for diabetes.

If you are a woman and have children, did you have high blood sugar during pregnancy? If so, you are at risk for diabetes. Pregnancy puts an added strain on the pancreatic beta cells. Because your own growing tissues and those of your developing fetus require increased amounts of energy, and because you must deposit fat in your own body for use during lactation, your body requires more insulin. If the beta cells are not able to keep up with these extra demands, insulin production will be insufficient and blood sugar will rise. If your blood sugar rises too high, you may require treatment during pregnancy. You have what we call gestational diabetes, and even if it disappears after delivery (it usually does), you are at risk for developing maturity-onset diabetes later in life. A higher-than-normal blood sugar during pregnancy that does not require treatment must also be considered a warning sign. If you fall into this category, you must also be considered at risk. If you don't know what your blood sugar was during pregnancy, ask your doctor who will have it on record. If you are pregnant now, ask your doctor if your blood sugar is normal. If it is, you need not worry about this risk factor. If it is high, at least you are aware that you are at high risk and will be able to do something about it after your infant is born.

Have you ever had an abnormal glucose tolerance test? A glucose tolerance test is performed by having a person drink a fixed amount of glucose (100 grams) in water, then doing blood-sugar determinations periodically for the next four to six hours. This test will determine the ability of the pancreatic islets to produce insulin. As the blood sugar rises from the initial loading dose, the beta cells respond by releasing insulin. This promptly results in a lowering of the blood sugar, which, in turn, signals the beta cells to cut back insulin production. If a person has a "tendency to diabetes," the beta cells respond sluggishly and the blood sugar rises initially to levels above normal. In addition, once the situation is brought under control by the release of insulin, and the blood sugar returns to normal, the sluggish beta cells are unable to respond normally and continue to release insulin beyond the necessary time. The result is that the blood sugar drops *below* normal before it returns to its proper range. This high one-hour blood-sugar level followed by a low three- or four-hour blood-

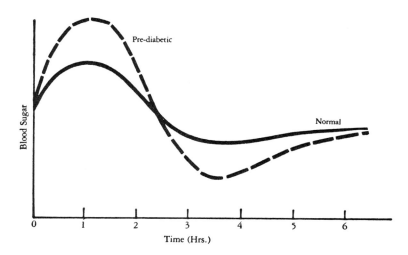

Pre-diabetic

Normal

Blood Sugar

0   1   2   3   4   5   6

Time (Hrs.)

sugar level is the characteristic diabetic or prediabetic pattern. Figure 3 compares diagrammatically a normal and a prediabetic glucose tolerance curve.

Glucose tolerance tests are performed by physicians for a variety of reasons. If you have had one, you should know if it was normal. If it was not normal, was it a prediabetic-type curve? If it was, you are at increased risk for developing diabetes.

While not as definitive as a glucose tolerance test, a high fasting blood-sugar level should alert you and your physician to the possibility of prediabetes, and you should then have a glucose tolerance test for more definitive data. Fasting blood sugars are easily done, inexpensive, and require at most the discomfort of a pricked finger. Anyone with a history of diabetes in the family or with any other risk factor for diabetes should have this test done as part of an annual physical examination.

Certain medications, the most important of which are the cortisonelike drugs, will raise blood-sugar levels independently and thereby invoke an insulin-releasing response in the pancreatic beta cells. A sluggish response by these cells will result in a "diabeticlike" syndrome, often called cortisone-induced diabetes. If you have been told that you respond in this manner, you are at increased risk for developing maturity-onset diabetes later in life. Any person who takes cortisone or its derivatives, particularly for a chronic illness such as asthma or arthritis, should have a glucose tolerance test or at least have a fasting blood sugar performed while under the influence of the drug. If a diabetic pattern emerges, it is a warning to take whatever steps are possible to lower your risk.

Finally, are you obese? The question of obesity as an *independent* risk factor for diabetes has not yet been settled. Certainly there is a strong association between obesity and maturity-onset diabetes. But both diseases have a strong genetic component; hence, it is possible that people who are genetically prone to diabetes are also genetically prone to obesity. However, a number of studies suggest that the relationship of diabetes to obesity is more than this type of genetic linking. First, as I have indicated, obesity puts a specific strain on the pancreatic islet cells. Second, in some obese patients who develop diabetes, weight reduction alone can control the disease. Third, in populations where diabetes was once rare, the disease has become much more common as that population has become heavier. These data strongly suggest that in people who are at risk for diabetes, obesity will significantly increase that risk. What is much less clear is whether obesity per se increases a person's risk for diabetes.

More people without any other known risk factors for diabetes develop the disease if they are obese than if they are lean. While this last fact does not prove that obesity is an *independent* risk factor for diabetes, it suggests that we treat it as if it were. Since we learned in the previous chapter that obesity should be prevented for many different reasons, I am going to include it as a risk factor for diabetes even if other risk factors are absent. From a practical standpoint, until more information is available I believe this is the most prudent course to take.

What about the lean individual with a sweet tooth? The person who consumes large amounts of refined sugar and does not gain weight? We all know and envy people like these. Are they increasing their risk for maturity-onset diabetes? If they have no other risk factors, they are probably not; if they are already at risk, we are not certain. There are theoretical reasons why consumption of large amounts of refined sugar might increase the stress on an already susceptible pancreas. However, there are no data suggesting that this actually occurs. Thus, we will assume that a person who has an increased risk for diabetes will not increase that risk further by consuming moderate amounts of refined sugar. As for the true "sugarholic," even though the evidence may not support my belief, I feel that the possibility of additionally increasing your risk is sufficiently strong that I recommend you reduce the amount of refined sugar in your diet.

Calculating Your Risk Score

Genetics
Since diabetes is genetic in origin, it will be more prevalent in some populations than in others. Blacks, Amerindians, and Jews of European extraction are among those who have a high incidence of the disease. But diabetes can and does occur in almost all groups. Therefore, you are not completely safe even if you belong to a low-risk group.

In the case of diabetes perhaps what is more important is your own family history. Plot your family health tree with great care. Question your living relatives about their health and that of their ancestors. Spread the branches as far as possible. If your relatives are not sure, try to piece together as much information as possible. Even if only one close relative has definitely had diabetes, your risk is increased. How much depends on how prevalent this disease is in your family health tree. If only one or two distant relatives have had diabetes, score 3; if a few close relatives or many more distant relatives are diabetics, score 5. If, in addition, you belong to a high-risk population, add 2.

Pregnancy

If during pregnancy you have been diagnosed as having gestational diabetes, score 5. If you have had persistently high blood-sugar levels or an abnormal glucose tolerance test during pregnancy, score 5. If your fasting blood sugar was elevated occasionally during pregnancy, score 3. If you have had one or more very large babies (nine pounds or more), score 2; this is because infants of mothers with diabetes or a tendency toward it are often large.

Abnormal Blood Sugars

If you have had a glucose tolerance test and it resulted in a diabeticlike curve or a higher-than-normal half-hour or one-hour blood sugar (even if the values were not high enough to diagnose diabetes) this significantly increases your risk for developing the disease, so score 5. If on several occasions your fasting blood sugar was high, you should have a glucose tolerance test performed. If it is abnormal, score 5. However, even if it is normal, you must consider yourself at increased risk if you show repeated high fasting blood-sugar levels—score 3.

Drug-Induced High Blood-Sugar Levels

Adrenal steroids are widely used in the treatment of a large number of chronic diseases and are consumed by many patients for long periods of time. As we have seen, these drugs independently raise blood-sugar levels, and insulin is called forth by these high levels. Thus, the beta cells of any patient consuming these drugs will be under constant stimulation. If you have a tendency toward diabetes, your beta cells may not respond perfectly and your blood sugar may be somewhat elevated. Any patient with steroid-induced high blood sugars should have a glucose tolerance test performed while on steroids. If a diabeticlike curve appears, score 5. If not, you cannot be complacent—score 3.

Obesity

If you are truly obese, that is, 120 percent or more of your ideal weight, you must consider yourself at high risk for diabetes even if you have no other risk factors. Therefore, I am assigning a risk factor of 5 to this condition. If you are overweight, but not frankly obese (105 to 120 percent of your ideal weight), score 3. Suppose you are not obese but are at high risk for becoming obese (see the previous chapter)—score 2.

Add up your score. If it totals 5 or more, you are at high enough risk to modify your diet so as to lower that risk.

Risk Factor	Maximum Score	Your Score
Family history	3–5	
High-risk population	2	
Gestational diabetes or repeated abnormal blood sugars during pregnancy	5	
Occasional abnormal blood sugars during pregnancy	3	
Abnormal glucose tolerance test	5	
Occasional high fasting blood sugar	3	
Cortisone-induced high blood sugar	5	
Frank obesity	5	
5–15% overweight	3	
High risk for obesity	2	
Total	36–38	

As you can see, being moderately overweight or being at risk for obesity in the absence of any other risk factor does not necessitate dietary modifications. By contrast, a strong family history of gestational diabetes, an abnormal glucose tolerance test, or frank obesity all place you in a high-risk category. Fill out the chart on page 121.

If your total score is 5 or more, you should attempt to lower your risk for diabetes.

Dietary Principles to Lower Your Risk for Diabetes

The overall dietary strategy we shall use will attempt to achieve two objectives simultaneously—first, to prevent or at least delay the occurrence of diabetes, and second, to prevent or at least minimize its complications if, as may happen, the disease does occur. The first objective is best achieved by controlling calories; the second by controlling fat. Let me explain the reasons behind this dietary approach.

As we have seen, the one major risk factor for diabetes which you can do something about is obesity. Thus, if you are obese it is important that you lose weight. If you are overweight (but not obese) and your total score is over 5, you should reduce to as close to your ideal weight as possible. If you are at risk for obesity and your total score is over 5, it is important that you do not become obese and therefore you must pay particular attention to controlling your weight.

In Chapter 4 I outlined the safest and in the long run the most effective way to lose weight and to keep it off. The same methods should be employed to lower your risk for diabetes. Since refined sugar is a food of very low nutrient density, large amounts of it should not be consumed on any reducing diet. This is especially true if a major reason for controlling your weight is to lower your risk for diabetes. If you are a true sugarholic, you may be putting an unnecessary strain on your beta cells, and you are surely consuming calories in an inefficient manner. Thus, while you need not avoid all sugar, you should cut back sufficiently to allow the rest of your low-calorie diet to provide all the essential nutrients you require.

In our society, a major principle of any reducing diet is lowering the consumption of fat. Fat is the most concentrated source of calories. Therefore, you get the maximum caloric benefit per gram of any food you eliminate from your diet if that food is high in fat. In a weight-control diet, it is even more important to minimize your risk for diabetes by restricting the amount of fat.

One of the major complications of diabetes is atherosclerosis, which may lead to heart attack and stroke. Consequently, a person who has diabetes is automatically at high risk for atherosclerosis (see Chapter 2). Similarly, someone at high risk for diabetes is potentially at high risk for atherosclerosis. Since many people who are at risk for diabetes will develop the disease even if they control their weight, it is important that both a low-calorie and a low-fat diet are introduced.

If you are destined to become diabetic, the earlier you begin to control your serum lipids, the better. A low-fat diet (particularly a low-saturated-fat diet) is the best way to do this. Chapter 2 outlines such a diet. It is by nature relatively low in calories; hence, if you are not obese, you may not need to control your caloric intake any further. If you are obese, use this diet and combine it with the principles outlined above; avoid empty calories such as alcohol and refined sugar; consume foods of high nutrient density; eat plenty of roughage (fiber); and increase your level of exercise. To construct your diet refer to Chapter 2. Remember, diabetes is a constant threat if you are at high risk. Thus, the program you will embark on is not a short-term reducing diet to drop five or ten pounds quickly. It is a lifelong eating pattern and must be approached as

such. Quick results are not important; it is a sustained reduction in weight and lowering of your serum lipids that
will give you maximum benefit.

Dietary Treatment of Diabetes

If you already have diabetes, controlling your diet will be
a major part of your treatment. If juvenile-onset diabetes
is the problem, you will also need insulin. By contrast,
maturity-onset diabetes may or may not require insulin
injections. In some cases, particularly if you are obese and
the disease is mild, weight reduction may be enough to
control the disease. The balanced low-calorie approach
remains best since it is most likely to produce long-term
results, and long-term results in a patient with diabetes are
essential. It may be more dangerous to lose weight and
gain it back several times than to remain obese, since such
"seesawing" may put stress on the beta cells of your pancreas even more than being obese does.

It is even more important that you limit your fat along
with your calories than it was in the preventive diet. If
you already have diabetes, you are automatically at risk
for atherosclerosis. Therefore, a low-total-fat, low-saturated-fat, low-cholesterol diet is necessary. Most individuals with maturity-onset diabetes will require insulin
injections. If you have diabetes, regardless of the type, and
need insulin, the foundation of your eating pattern similarly will be the low-calorie, low-fat diet. This diet will almost certainly be high in carbohydrate, which is good.
Contrary to what you may have been told a high-carbohydrate diet is preferable for anyone with diabetes. Some
interesting statistics highlight this fact. Until recently in this
country, most people with diabetes were treated with a
low-carbohydrate diet, which was high in protein and in
fat. In Japan, diabetes was treated with the standard Japanese high-carbohydrate diet. The mortality rate from the

most serious complication of diabetes, atherosclerosis, was much higher in the United States than in Japan. The same disease, the same type of insulin treatment—the only difference was the type of diet used. The high-carbohydrate diet gave the lower mortality figures. Today, we follow the principle that insulin controls the disease; diet lowers the risk of certain major complications.

Although the basic diet for any diabetic is a high-carbohydrate, low-fat diet, the nature of the carbohydrate consumed may be very important. If you are being treated with insulin, you will be taking one or more injections during the day. The type of insulin prescribed by your physician may vary. Some are long acting, others are short acting. You may be taking either type, or more often, a combination of both. The insulin is given in such a manner as to reach its peak concentration in your blood at the same time your blood-sugar level reaches its highest value. In addition, it is given in a dose designed to bring that blood sugar back to normal without producing hypoglycemia. Thus, whereas your own beta cells *react* to your blood-sugar level, when the cells do not function properly, your doctor must *anticipate* the level of your blood sugar when he prescribes insulin for you.

You can make your doctor's job easier, and hence bring your diabetes under control better, by following two additional dietary rules. The first is consistency—you must try to consume the same number of calories at the same times during the day. This does not mean that every day you must eat the same number of calories at every meal and every snack exactly at the same time. What it means is that you and your physician will work out an eating pattern that is consistent with your needs and with your life-style, and you will tailor the time and dose of your insulin accordingly. This pattern may be more difficult to follow on weekends than on weekdays; it may be different when you are on vacation; it may change somewhat on days when you are physically very active. For example, during the week, when you go to work you may consume 25 percent of your calories at breakfast, 20 percent at lunch, 30 percent at dinner, and split the remaining 25 percent between two snacks, one in midmorning and one in midevening. By contrast, on weekends you may consume 40 percent of your calories at brunch, 40 percent at dinner, and the remaining 20 percent as snacks. The timing of your insulin dose may be different, but either pattern can be dealt with effectively. After a while with your doctor's approval you may be able to alter your anticipated eating and activity schedule. Although this approach may seem very restrictive, it really is not. Most people establish routine patterns in the way they eat and vary them very little. The standard pattern of breakfast, coffee break, lunch, dinner, and evening snack is followed by millions of Americans. Sure, these people can change more easily than you can, but this is a price you must pay to keep your diabetes under proper control.

The second dietary rule concerns the nature of the carbohydrate you consume. Carbohydrate comes in two forms, simple sugars, consisting of a single molecule (monosaccharides) or two molecules joined together (disaccharides); or complex carbohydrates, consisting of many simple sugars joined together as a chain or a series of branches. The simple sugars are rapidly absorbed from the intestines and reach the bloodstream very soon after they are consumed. Therefore, your blood sugar will increase sharply if you consume a large quantity of simple sugars. The complex carbohydrates fall into two groups: those that are slowly broken down into simple sugars and then absorbed into the bloodstream (starches), and those that are not broken down and pass out of your body intact in the stool (fiber). Thus, dietary starch gives your body a low but steady source of glucose, and dietary fiber does not affect your blood sugar at all.

A good diet for a person with diabetes derives most of its carbohydrate calories from starches while restricting

TABLE 12

	Typical American Diet	*Recommended Diabetic Diet*
Carbohydrate	40% (high in simple sugars)	50%–60% (high in complex carbohydrates, e.g. starches and vegetables)
Fat	40% (high in saturated fat)	20%–30% (1:1:1 ratio of polyunsaturated to monounsaturated to saturated fat)
Protein	20%	20%
Fiber	low	high

the amount of simple sugar. There is some evidence that keeping your blood sugar within a narrow range may have a beneficial effect on some of the other complications of diabetes. Besides atherosclerosis and its accompanying heart disease and stroke, which are known as macrovascular complications (or diseases of the *large* blood vessels), the most serious are called microvascular complications (or diseases of the *small* blood vessels). These complications are serious because the small blood vessels most often involved are those in the kidney and in the retina of the eye. This is why severe kidney disease and blindness are such dreaded complications of diabetes. Recent evidence suggests that the more stable your dietary control, the lower the incidence of microvascular complications. A careful diet may lower your risk not only for atherosclerosis, but for kidney and eye disease as well.

Table 12 outlines the nutrient content of the typical American diet, and compares it with the ideal diet for a person with diabetes.

Let me summarize the most important nutritional guidelines for a person suffering from diabetes:

- Calories should be aimed at achieving ideal weight. (In the juvenile diabetic, this often means gaining weight; in the maturity-onset diabetic, this usually means losing weight.)
- Fat should be limited to 20 to 30 percent of the total calories consumed.
- Saturated fat should supply 10 to 15 percent of the total calories, and vegetable fat (polyunsaturated and monounsaturated) should provide the other 10 to 15 percent.
- Protein can range from 12 to 24 percent of all calories (not critical).
- Simple sugars should be kept to 10 to 15 percent of all calories consumed, and only a small amount should come from refined sugars.
- The remainder of the calories (around 40 percent) should come from complex carbohydrate (starch).
- Dietary fiber should be increased by ingesting raw vegetables and whole-grain and bran cereals.

This last recommendation is made because several recent studies have demonstrated that adding 20 grams of crude fiber to the diets of diabetic patients reduced their blood-sugar levels and the amount of insulin necessary to maintain good control of the disease. There are several possible explanations for these results. The one that seems to have the most support currently is that fiber delays the absorption of simple sugars from the gastrointestinal tract. For example, dietary fiber might delay emptying of the stomach, thereby slowing entrance of the meal into the small intestine, where absorption must take place. Alternatively, dietary fiber may affect the cells that are responsible for breaking down and absorbing simple sugars, and therefore might help slow glucose absorption.

Whatever the exact mechanism, the result is a slower and more sustained release of glucose from the gastrointestinal tract into the bloodstream. We have seen that this is very desirable, since it will prevent the wide swings in blood sugar that may occur when simple sugars are ingested in the absence of fiber. In addition, it often reduces the amount of insulin necessary to control blood sugar.

From a practical standpoint, a person with diabetes should consume natural sugars in a form as close to the natural state as possible. For example, an apple is better than applesauce or apple juice. In addition, there is no reason why a diabetic individual should not increase the fiber content of his or her regular diet, or even add fiber to the diet in the form of bran or raw vegetables.

Although the importance of fiber in the diet of the diabetic patient has become more and more firmly established, the issue of the rate of release of simple sugars from complex carbohydrate foods is far from determined. Recent studies in which different foods were tested revealed some surprising results when speeds were compared at which one food or another raises the blood-sugar levels. A system, currently being evaluated, lists foods in their "glucose equivalents." Glucose is assigned the number one hundred and other foods are compared with it. Foods can then be related to each other as a percentage of the rate of absorption of glucose. This number is called the glycemic index. The lower the number, the more slowly the food raises the blood sugar. Table 13 shows the glycemic indexes for a number of common foods. Notice that certain foods previously thought to affect the blood sugar very slowly actually have a *higher* glycemic index than refined sugar (sucrose). Carrots, potatoes, and certain breads and cereals fall into this category.

It is too early to say whether a person with diabetes should avoid those foods with high glycemic indexes. However, I am sure that in the next few years we will be able to pinpoint those foods which raise blood sugar very rapidly. This will undoubtedly influence our dietary rec-

TABLE 13   Glycemic Indexes of Certain Common
Carbohydrate Foods

	Glycemic index (%)		*Glycemic index (%)*
Grain, Cereal Products		Potato (instant)	80
		Potato (new)	70
Bread (white)	69	Potato (sweet)	48
Bread (whole grain)	72	Rutabaga*	72
		Yams	51
Buckwheat	51		
Millet	71	*Dried and Canned Legumes*	
Pastry	59		
Rice (brown)	66	Beans (canned, baked)	40
Rice (white)	72	Beans (butter)	36
Spaghetti (whole-wheat)	42	Beans (green)	31
		Beans (kidney)	29
Spaghetti (white)	50	Beans (soya)	15
Spongecake	46	Beans (canned soya)	14
Sweet corn	59	Peas (blackeye)	33
		Peas (chick)	36
Breakfast Cereals		Peas (green)	47
All-Bran	51	Lentils	29
Cornflakes	80		
Granola	66	*Fruits*	
Oatmeal	49	Apples (Golden Delicious)	39
Shredded Wheat	67		
		Bananas	62
Cookies, Crackers		Orange juice	46
Digestive	59	Oranges	40
Oatmeal	54	Raisins	64
Water	63		
		Sugars	
Fresh Legumes		Fructose	20
Broad beans*	79	Glucose	100
Frozen peas	51	Maltose	105
		Sucrose	59
Root Vegetables			
Beets*	64	*Dairy Products*	
Carrots*	92	Ice cream	36
Parsnips*	97	Milk (skim)	32

	Glycemic index (%)		Glycemic index (%)
Dairy Products		Mars bar	68
Milk (whole)	34	Peanuts*	13
Yogurt	36	Potato chips	51
		Sausages	28
Miscellaneous		Tomato soup	38
Fish sticks	38		
Honey	87		

*Only 25 g carbohydrate portion given

ommendations regarding the treatment of some diabetic patients.

Finally, in addition to the composition of the diet, the frequency of meals is extremely important, particularly in the juvenile-onset diabetic, but also in some patients with severe maturity-onset diabetes. As we have seen, wide swings in the level of blood sugar are best avoided. To accomplish this, your physician will probably use a combination of long-acting and short-acting insulin. Spacing your meals will help by producing a lower but more sustained elevation of blood sugar throughout the day. The person with juvenile-onset diabetes or severe insulin-dependent maturity-onset diabetes should consume five or even six meals during the day. A good routine would be to have breakfast, a midmorning snack, lunch, a late-afternoon snack, dinner, and an evening snack shortly before retiring.

How to Choose the Proper Foods

The diet I am recommending to lower your risk for diabetes if your score is above 5 depends on whether you are overweight. For those of you who are obese, the diet discussed in Chapter 4 should be instituted. There is no difference between weight-reduction diets for a person at risk for diabetes and for a person who is not. However, the urgency of starting weight reduction may be considerably greater if you are obese and are at high risk for diabetes. If you are, I hope that you do not procrastinate. The time for beginning your reducing diet is now.

If you are at risk for diabetes (whether you are overweight or not), you should use the Prudent Diet (low-total-fat, low-saturated fat, low-cholesterol) outlined in Chapter 2. It is a low-cost insurance policy that should be taken out by anyone at risk for diabetes. In addition, if one of your risk factors is obesity or a tendency toward it, you should institute necessary calorie control as outlined in Chapter 4.

In addition, the diabetic individual should lower the amount of refined sugar in the diet, introduce day-to-day consistency, and proper meal spacing. All these can be accomplished and still provide you with plenty of variety in your food choices.

Calculating Your Diabetic Diet

Find your ideal body weight on the table on page 77. Because most food calculations use the metric system, convert your ideal body weight from pounds to kilograms by dividing the number by 2.2.

Now, calculate the amount of energy you need per day for each kilogram of ideal body weight, depending on your actual body weight and your level of physical activity. Use the chart below:

	Sedentary	Moderately active	Extremely active
		Calories per kilogram	
Overweight	20–25	30	35
Normal	30	35	40
Underweight	35	40	45–50

Let us assume your ideal weight is 160 pounds. Dividing this figure by 2.2 gives about 73 kilograms. If you are obese and lead a sedentary life, multiply your ideal weight (73 kilograms) by 20; 1,460 calories per day is what you should consume. If you are overweight but not obese, multiply your ideal weight (73 kilograms) by 25; 1,765 calories per day is what you are allowed.

By contrast, if you are a very active person whose ideal weight is 73 kilograms and who is not overweight, multiply 73 by 40; you should consume almost 3,000 calories per day. Let us take as a final example a tall, somewhat underweight young juvenile diabetic who should weigh 160 pounds (73 kilograms) and who takes part in competitive athletics. Such an individual might require 73 times 50, or 3,650 calories per day.

Having determined the number of calories you require, you are now ready to divide those calories into protein, carbohydrate, and fat.

Protein

Your protein requirement is about 1.5 grams per kilogram of your ideal weight, no matter what you actually weigh. Thus, all the individuals described above would have the same protein requirement—73 times 1.5, or about 110 grams. This represents 440 calories. The obese, sedentary individual will therefore be taking in 30 percent of his calories as protein. This amount is somewhat high, but is acceptable if he has no kidney disease. However, if your protein intake represents as high a percentage of your calories as this, check with your physician; he or she may wish to lower it a little. The other two individuals should have no problems with this amount of protein, 440 calories representing about 15 percent of one's total calories and about 12 percent for the other, the very active underweight diabetic; both amounts are adequate but not excessive.

Carbohydrate

Carbohydrate should account for 50 to 60 percent of total calories—about 750 calories for the obese and sedentary person, 900 calories for the overweight sedentary person, 1,600 calories for the active, not obese person, and 1,900 calories for the young, active underweight diabetic. Remember, only 10 to 15 percent of total calories should come from simple sugar and only a small amount of this should be refined sugar. Thus, the first person is allowed 150 calories from these carbohydrates, the second 200 calories, the third 300 calories, and the fourth 400 calories. More specifically then, the obese sedentary person can consume 600 calories as complex carbohydrate and 150 calories as simple sugar (total 750); the overweight sedentary person can consume 700 calories as complex carbohydrate and 200 as simple sugar (total 900); the normal-weight, very active person can consume 1,300 calories as complex carbohydrate and 300 as simple sugar (total 1,600); and the underweight diabetic athlete can take in 1,500 calories as complex carbohydrate and 400 as simple sugar (total 1,900).

Fat

The rest of your calories will come from fat. In the case of the first person discussed above, 1,460 (total) minus 440 (protein) and 750 (carbohydrate), or 270 calories will come from fat. One-half this amount (135 calories) should be saturated fat, and one-half, unsaturated fat. The second person could take in slightly more fat calories, 420; the third, about 1,000 calories; and the fourth, about 1,250 calories. Remember, protein and carbohydrate yield 4 calories per gram, whereas fat yields 9 calories per gram. Thus, even the young underweight athlete will be consuming only about 150 grams (about 5 ounces) of fat.

I have gone through these calculations to show you how diets for diabetics are created. For you to use these calculations to construct your own diet, you need to know the actual composition of all the foods you use. However, it is not practical for a diabetic to calculate his or her diet from scratch. Therefore, a simple method has been devised which uses exchange lists of foods containing similar nutrient contents. By knowing the number of calories you require and employing these exchange lists, you can put together a diet that meets all the criteria outlined above and offers at the same time a great deal of variety.

Using the exchange lists in Table 14 you can convert your diet requirements into food servings, and distribute these among three meals plus extra snacks without going through all the calculations.

The foods in the exchange lists are grouped according to their nutrient similarities: vegetables; fruits and juices; and starchy foods (breads, cereals, beans) are together as are meat, fish, and poultry; milk products; and fats. Within each list, foods are shown in specific quantities or units. The term "exchange" is used because a serving of a food within a list can be exchanged for another one within the same list. For example, on the fruit list you can exchange ten cherries for one-half cup of orange juice, if you prefer. On the meat list, you can substitute one ounce of lean beef for one ounce of fish or skinned poultry, or for two teaspoons of peanut butter. Or you can make two or more exchanges. For example, ten cherries and one-half cup of orange juice equal one apple (each equals one-half apple). Three meat exchanges would equal three ounces of lean meat, or three small lobster tails, or three-fourths of a cup of tunafish or salmon, or two eggs and one-half ounce of hard cheese. The possible combinations really leave a great deal of choice and allow for individual preferences.

The same exchange lists are used no matter how many calories you will be consuming. Table 15 lists the number of items from each exchange list permitted daily for persons taking in 1,000, 1,200, 1,500, and 1,800 calories (most adult-onset diabetics). If you need more calories, simply

TABLE 14*

List 1. Free Foods

Bouillon
Clear broth
Coffee
Tea
Gelatin, unsweet-
ened
Lemon, lime

Mustard
Pickle, sour
Pickle, dill—un-
sweetened
Vinegar
Chicory
Chinese cabbage

Endive
Escarole
Lettuce (all kinds)
Parsley
Radishes
Watercress

List 2. Vegetable Exchanges = ½ cup cooked or 1 cup raw

One exchange of vegetables contains about 5 grams of carbohydrate, 2 grams of protein, and 25 kcal.

Asparagus
Bean sprouts
Beans (green or
wax)
Broccoli
Beets
Brussels sprouts
Cabbage (all
kinds)
Carrots
Catsup (2 tbsp.)

Cauliflower
Celery
Cucumbers
Eggplant
Mushrooms
Okra
Onions
Peppers (red or
green)
Rutabaga

Sauerkraut
Summer squash
Tomatoes—1 cup
raw
½ cup cooked
Tomato or vegeta-
ble juice—6
oz.
All leafy greens

List 3. Fruit Exchanges

One exchange of fruit contains 10 grams of carbohydrate and
40 kcal.

FRUITS:
Apple—½ med.
Applesauce—½
cup
Apricots, fresh—2
med.
Apricots, dried—4
halves
Bananas—½ small
Blueberries—½
cup

Cantaloupe—¼
med. (6"
diam.)
Cherries—10 large
Dates—2
Figs, dried—1 small
Fruit cocktail,
canned—
½ cup

Grapefruit—½
small
Grapes—12
Honeydew
melon—⅓
(7" diam.)
Mango—½ small
Nectarine—1 small
Orange—1 small
Papaya—⅓ med.

FRUITS:
Peach—1 med.
Pear—1 small
Pineapple—½ cup
Prunes, dried—2
Raisins—2 tbsp.
Strawberries—¾
  cup

Tangerine—1 large
Watermelon—1
  cup, cubed

JUICES:
Apple, pineapple—
  ⅓ cup

Grapefruit, or-
  ange—½ cup
Grape, prune—¼
  cup

List 4. Starch Exchanges (cooked servings)

One exchange of starch contains 15 grams of carbohydrate, 2 grams of protein, and 70 kcal.

BREADS:
Any loaf—1 slice
Bagel—½
Dinner roll—1 (2"
  diam.)
English muffin—½
Bun, hamburger or
  hot dog—½
Cornbread
  (1½")—1
  cube
Tortilla (6"
  diam.)—1

VEGETABLES:
Beans or peas
  (plain),
  cooked—½
  cup
Corn—⅓ cup or
  ½ med. ear

Parsnips—⅔ cup
Potatoes, white—1
  small or ½ cup
Potatoes, sweet or
  yams—¼ cup
Pumpkin—¾ cup
Winter squash—½
  cup

CRACKERS:
Graham (2½"
  sq.)—2
Matzoh (4" × 6")—
  ½
Melba toast—4
Oyster (½ cup)—
  20
Pretzels—8 rings
RyKrisp—3

Saltines—5

CEREALS:
Hot cereal—½
  cup
Dry flakes—⅔ cup
Dry puffed—1½
  cups
Bran—5 tbsp.
Wheat germ—2
  tbsp.
Pasta—½ cup
Rice—½ cup

DESSERTS:
Fat-free sherbet—4
  oz.
Angel cake—1½"
  square

List 5. Meat Exchanges (cooked weight)

One exchange of lean meat contains 7 grams of protein, 3 grams of fat, and 55 kcal.

Beef, dried,
  chipped—1
  oz.

Beef, lamb, pork,
  veal, *lean
  only*—1 oz.

Cottage cheese,
  uncreamed—
  ¼ cup

TABLE 14 (*Continued*)

Poultry without skin—1 oz.	Tuna, packed in water—¼ cup	Egg—1 med.
Fish—1 oz.	Salmon, pink, canned—¼ cup	Hard cheese—½ oz.
Lobster—1 small tail		Peanut butter—2 tsp.
Oysters, clams, shrimp—5 med.		

List 6. *Milk Exchanges*

One exchange of milk contains 12 grams of carbohydrate, 8 grams of protein, and 80 kcal.

| Buttermilk, fat free—1 cup | Skim milk—1 cup | 1% fat milk—7 oz. |
| Yogurt, plain, made with nonfat milk—¾ cup | | |

List 7. *Fat Exchanges*

One exchange of fat contains 5 grams of fat and 45 kcal.

Avocado (4" diam.)—⅛	Mayonnaise—1 tsp.	Oil—1 tsp.
Bacon, crisp—1 slice	Roquefort dressing—2 tsp.	Olives—5 small
Butter, margarine—1 tsp.	Thousand Island dressing—2 tsp.	Peanuts—10
French dressing—1 tbsp.		Walnuts—6 small

Nutrition & Health (Diabetes), vol. 4, no. 4, 1982, pp. 3 and 4.

double the items in the appropriate column. For example, if you require 2,000 calories, double the 1,000-calorie list; if 3,000, double the 1,500-calorie list, and so forth.

When Table 15 is used, the protein intake at all calorie levels will be adequate, and vitamin and mineral supplementation should not be necessary if selections are made

TABLE 15*

List	Number of Portions Allowed for Various Calorie Levels			
	1000 Calories	1200 Calories	1500 Calories	1800 Calories
List 1—Free Foods	.... Unlimited			
List 2—Vegetable Exchanges	2	2	2	2
List 3 —Fruit Exchanges	3	3	3	3
List 4—Starch Exchanges	3	5	7	9
List 5—Protein Exchanges	6	6	7	7
List 6—Milk Exchanges	2	2	2	3
List 7—Fat Exchanges	2	2	6	7

*Nutrition & Health (Diabetes), vol. 4, no. 4, 1982, p. 5.

from a variety of foods, except that iron should be given to women on 1,000 or 1,200 calories.

Let us now actually construct a daily menu for a person on a 1,500-calorie diet.

By using similar menus that fit the overall number of exchanges listed in Table 15, you can devise an endless variety and still remain within the limitations set forth in this chapter. This system takes into account your individual food preferences, and when spaced according to your doctor's orders, it will allow the use of the minimum amount of insulin necessary to control your diabetes.

Since diabetes is often accompanied by other medical problems that require special diets, the basic diet may have to be further modified. Salt restriction may be necessary if you have heart or kidney disease. Some people with kidney or liver problems may need to lower their protein intake. Your doctor will advise you if additional dietary modifications are necessary. For most diabetic people, however, the basic diet offers calorie control, low fat, high complex carbohydrate, and low simple sugar, and if used wisely can provide ample amounts of fiber and plenty of variety. Remember, once you have diabetes, you will have it for the rest of your life; therefore, it is important to plan

Basic Plan*	Sample Menu	Free Foods
Morning		
List 3 = 1	½ small grapefruit	coffee, artificial
List 5 = 1	1 medium egg	sweetener
List 4 = 2	1 slice whole wheat bread & 1½ cup puffed cereal	
List 7 = 1	1 tsp. margarine	
List 6 = 1	1 cup (8 oz.) skim milk	
Noon		
List 5 = 2	½ cup tuna (in water)	lettuce, pickles,
List 4 = 2	2 slices bread	lemon juice,
List 7 = 3	2 tsp. mayonnaise & 1 tsp. oil	vinegar
List 2 = 1	3 slices tomato	
List 3 = 1	½ cup diced pineapple	
Evening		
List 2 = 1	½ cup string beans	lettuce, radishes,
List 5 = 4	4 oz. chicken (no skin)	soy sauce,
List 4 = 2	½ cup mashed potato & 4 oz. fat-free sherbet	parsley
List 7 = 2	2 tsp. margarine	
List 3 = 1	2 dates	
Snack		
List 6 = 1	8 oz. skim milk	coffee
List 4 = 1	1½ in. square sponge cake	

Nutrition & Health (Diabetes), vol. 4, no. 4, 1982, p. 5.

a diet that will offer you the most options. It may be difficult at first to use these lists, but in the long run it will be worth it.

By now, no doubt, you have noticed that this diet, though somewhat more restrictive than some, can be used not only for the person who already has diabetes but also by anyone who wishes to lose weight or lower his or her risk for atherosclerosis. It is not very different from the diets used in the chapters that discuss those diseases, and therefore it offers a viable alternative to people at risk for obesity or atherosclerosis. By contrast, this diet does not control your salt intake. If you are at risk for high blood pressure, this diet must be adjusted to your proper salt level in the same way as any other diet (see Chapter 3). Any person who has a combined high risk for diabetes and high blood pressure can modify this diet to lower its salt content and still get all the necessary nutrients.

Chapter 6

Cancer

It has been estimated that 50 percent of all types of cancer in women and 30 percent in men are associated with environmental factors. Of those factors, food supply is one of the most important. Recently, concern has been mounting that food additives of various kinds may be contributing to the rising incidence of certain types of cancer. Such commonly added materials as saccharin, red dye #2, and nitrites have all been implicated. In addition, there is mounting evidence that substances "contaminating" our food supply, such as pesticide residues or industrial waste products, are also increasing the risk of certain cancers. Even radioactive materials, like iodine 131 or strontium 90, turn up from time to time in our food supply.

These data, important as they are, should not be allowed to detract from another aspect of the problem of diet and cancer—that there is a strong association between the kinds of food we eat and the increasing incidence of specific types of cancer. This problem, which may be more difficult to deal with since it defies regulation, cannot be laid at the feet of any one product or group of manufacturers. The evidence comes both from studies of large human populations and from experiments on animals. The best data have been collected with two extremely common types of cancer—those of the breast and colon.

Breast Cancer

Cancer of the breast is the most common cancer striking American women and a leading cause of death in the United States. In other countries, however, the incidence of breast cancer is much lower. If we list countries in the order of incidence of breast cancer, we can make an important generalization, with certain specific exceptions. The more highly developed the country, the higher the incidence of breast cancer. More careful scrutiny of the data gives us certain clues as to what aspect of "modern living" contributes to this problem, as certain westernized countries—for example, Japan—do not show this high incidence of breast cancer.

By contrast, when Japanese people migrate to California, their children have the same incidence of this cancer as other Californians if they adopt a western eating pattern. If, on the other hand, they continue to eat as their parents did in Japan, relatively few have cancer of the breast. Therefore, it is some element in our western diet that contributes to the high incidence of the disease. The strongest correlation appears to be with the amount of fat the diet contains. The more fat the population of a particular country consumes, the higher the incidence of breast cancer, regardless of how developed a country is. The United States, with its high-fat diet, ranks high, but certain countries that consume more fat, such as Finland, rank even higher.

How does this high consumption of fat contribute to breast cancer? We know from other studies and from the fact that the disease occurs far more commonly in women than in men that hormones play an important role. Animal studies suggest that a diet high in fat will result in an imbalance of at least two hormones, and it is postulated that this hormone imbalance in some way promotes the

occurrence of cancer of the breast. Women who consume a relatively high-fat diet may alter their hormonal
balance and by so doing become more susceptible to developing breast cancer.

Colon Cancer

Colon cancer (cancer of the large intestine) is very common in the United States, and its incidence is increasing.
Like cancer of the breast, it occurs more frequently in developed countries, and certain migrating populations
demonstrate an incidence of this cancer that more closely
matches that of their adopted country as soon as they
change their eating patterns to resemble those of the
native population. The best correlation of cancer of the
colon is with dietary fat. Figure 4 demonstrates this
correlation. The more fat consumed, the higher the incidence of the disease. Particular groups in the United States
who for various reasons consume relatively little fat, such
as Seventh Day Adventists, show a low incidence of colon
cancer.

Unlike breast cancer, colon cancer occurs with equal
frequency in men and women. So, sex hormones play little or no role in its development. How then does this disease occur? While we are not yet sure, animal experiments
suggest that a high-fat diet changes the normal bacterial
makeup of the large intestine in such a way as to favor the
survival of bacteria that can easily transform the fat into
other products. One or more products of this bacterial
transformation may act as a carcinogen (cancer-produc-
ing agent) or may promote the activity of carcinogens already present in the large intestine. For example, certain
substances normally secreted into the intestine in the bile
are known to be carcinogens. It is thought that a high-fat
diet may indirectly increase the carcinogenic activity of
these substances. In addition, there are data which sug-

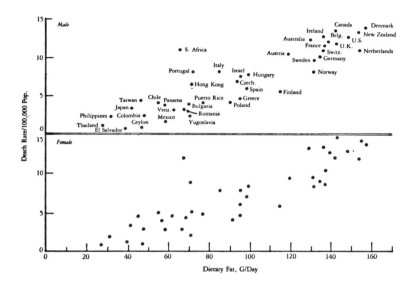

FIGURE 4. Correlation between the consumption of dietary fat and mortality from cancer of the colon.

gest that the low-fiber content in the American diet may further aggravate the problem.

Fiber is that portion of the carbohydrate within our food which is not digested and absorbed by our bodies. It is derived from plant sources, such as the bran of certain grains, and from the skin and fleshy portion of certain fruits and vegetables. Dietary fiber will draw water into it; hence, as the fiber passes through the gastrointestinal tract, it will soften the stool. The softer the stool, the faster it is propelled through the large intestine (colon) and the less time it is in contact with the intestinal wall. Thus, the wall of the colon will not be exposed to any cancer-inducing component in the stool for as long a time if the diet is high in fiber. It is theorized that this is the mechanism by which a high-fiber diet protects against colon cancer.

Uterine Cancer

Cancer of the uterus, one of the most common forms of the disease in women, is slightly more frequent in obese women than in lean women. This is particularly true in women who have been obese since childhood. In one study, uterine cancer was found to be one and a half times as frequent in women who suffered from obesity since adolescence than in women who were not obese. This is just one more reason to avoid obesity, particularly the adolescent form, which often leads to an intractable form of adult obesity.

Other Cancers

Although the data are by no means as complete as with cancer of the breast or colon, there is some evidence that cancer of the ovaries and of the prostate may also be directly related to dietary fat intake. Cancer of the stomach, while undoubtedly related to dietary factors, is probably not related to dietary fat. This cancer is much more prevalent in Japan than in the United States and its incidence decreases when Japanese people migrate to California or Hawaii. However, it has been pointed out that the incidence of stomach cancer in Japan is decreasing and that this may be caused not by changes in dietary factors per se but by the increased use of refrigeration as opposed to salting to preserve foods. Thus, the problem of discovering the causes of the various kinds of cancer is very complicated, and studying general trends in food intake can sometimes be misleading.

Determining Your Risk

Cancer of the Breast
Cancer of the breast occurs almost exclusively in women; the risk in men is so small that the male population can be excluded from any subsequent discussion. Within the female population, however, certain other factors can increase your risk.

Your Race
Cancer of the breast is most common among Caucasian women, less common among black women, and least common among Oriental women.

Family History
A strong family history increases your risk for breast cancer. The closer the member of your family tree who has or had the disease, the higher the risk. If your mother had breast cancer your chances of developing it are statistically greater than if your great-aunt or a cousin had the disease. If the disease appears regularly in your family tree, your risk is greater than if it appears sporadically. For this reason, any woman who wants to determine her risk for breast cancer should examine her family health tree as carefully and completely as possible.

Socioeconomic Status
There is evidence that regardless of other risk factors, women of high socioeconomic status, or, as it is sometimes referred to, high social status, are at slightly higher risk than women of lower social or economic status. The exact reason for this is not known, but most researchers

feel that it is due to differences in diet, and probably to the higher amounts of fat consumed by the higher-status women.

Marital Status
Single women are at greater risk than married women. This may be because they are much less likely to have completed a pregnancy and, as we shall see, the more pregnancies a woman has undergone, the lower her risk.

The Number of Pregnancies (Parity)
The more times a woman has become pregnant and carried to term, the *lower* her risk for cancer of the breast. While there is some reduction in risk associated with each subsequent pregnancy, the greatest difference is between women who have never carried a pregnancy to term and those who have completed at least one pregnancy.

Age at First Completed Pregnancy
The younger you are when you complete your first pregnancy, the lower your risk for breast cancer. The major increase occurs in women who are over thirty-five at the time they complete their first pregnancy. It is important to note that this is no reason not to have your first child later in life because the increase in risk is very small. Deciding not to have a child will also *increase* your risk, since women who have never carried a pregnancy to term are at increased risk.

Menstruation
The earlier your menstrual period started (menarche), the greater your risk for breast cancer. Women who reached puberty late are at lower risk than those who underwent an early puberty. The trend toward earlier puberty in girls in western countries may be associated with the increasing incidence of breast cancer. There is some evidence that this trend toward earlier menarche is associated with a

"better" diet. Some epidemiologic studies suggest that to the extent that this "better" diet is higher in fat, it may be contributing to the increased incidence of breast cancer. Japanese girls attain puberty later than American girls. The average caloric intake of the Japanese diet is about 1,000 calories less than in our diet. The difference is primarily in the amount of fat consumed. The Japanese eat far less fat than we do. There is evidence which suggests that the heavier a girl is, the earlier her menstrual periods will occur. As Japanese girls in higher socioeconomic classes have adopted western life-styles and a western diet, their average weight has increased, their dietary fat consumption has gone up, their menstrual periods have begun earlier, and their incidence of breast cancer has risen. Thus, the increased risk imparted by the early onset of menstruation may be indirect. The direct cause may be an increase in the fat content of the diet.

Menopause
The later the occurrence of menopause, the longer your reproductive life, the higher your risk of developing cancer of the breast. This increased risk is because breast cancer is related to the hormonal differences between men and women, and these hormonal differences are greatest during a woman's reproductive life. Thus, women who have shorter reproductive lives because of late onset of menarche, early menopause occurring naturally or induced artificially, or both, are at lower risk than women who have long reproductive lives.

Cancer of the Uterus
The risk factors for cancer of the uterus are much less well defined than those for cancer of the breast. One risk factor seems to be obesity, especially a history of it during adolescence. This increased risk is relatively small and may be indirect. Obesity is associated with early menarche, and it is possible that it is this combination of factors that may

contribute to the increased risk. Other factors that increase risk somewhat are late menopause or the use of estrogens to prevent menopause. The latter is a major risk factor, but as we shall see in the chapter on osteoporosis, the use of progesterone together with estrogen substantially reduces and may even eliminate the risk.

Cancer of the Colon

No general risk factors for cancer of the colon have been defined clearly enough to separate people at high or low risk. There is, however, at least one specific risk factor which, if present, should be under a physician's management: polyps. Polyps are noncancerous growths that may occur singly or in groups within the intestine. The existence of polyps under certain conditions predisposes individuals to colon cancer and they may therefore have to be removed.

Scoring Your Risk

Even for cancer of the breast, which has the best-defined risk factors, it is not possible, nor would it be helpful at this stage of our knowledge, to construct a meaningful scoring system that would separate individuals who are at high risk from those at low or moderate risk. Certainly, if you have several of the risk factors mentioned, your risk is increased. Cancer of the breast is serious enough that all women should consider dietary modification, especially if they have one or more risk factors. Since neither cancer of the colon nor uterine cancer can be scored, and since the dietary modifications are similar to those needed to reduce the risk of breast cancer, instituting a low-fat, high-fiber diet will give you protection against those diet-related cancers, which occur with some frequency in this country.

What then is the answer? Certainly there is enough evidence to encourage prudence in the amount of fat we eat. As pointed out in the Introduction, Americans consume far too much fat. Someday we may be able to identify specific individuals who are at risk of contracting particular cancers and therefore will be able to recommend dietary changes designed especially for them. At present, however, we can only recommend dietary changes based on the statistical chances of developing certain cancers.

A High-Fiber, Low-Fat Diet

The amount of fiber recommended in this diet is 15 grams per day. At present, it is estimated that most Americans consume 4 to 6 grams daily, compared with 25 to 30 grams eaten by more primitive people. Fiber-rich foods are fruits, vegetables, peas, beans, nuts, and grains. In general, these foods are also sources of complex carbohydrate (starches) and, except for nuts, are very low in fat.

On the other hand, whole milk and whole-milk products, red meats, fats, oils and dressings, pastries, and desserts are high in fat and virtually fiber-free. Ideally, fat, whether visible (as in meat) or invisible (as in cheese), should contribute no more than 25 percent of the day's total calories. If you eat 2,000 calories a day, no more than 500 should come from fat, and that amount is equal to 55 grams of fat. To keep within that amount, fried foods and spreads are discouraged and low-fat protein foods are encouraged (see Table 16).

Making the recommended changes means making rather simple adjustments. Eat more vegetables—the more raw the better—and whole-grain products. Eat the skin on your boiled or baked potato; consider raisins or almonds as alternatives to candy bars; and avoid fried foods in favor of fresh fruits and salads.

A diet high in fiber and low in fat is enjoyed by people all over the world. People who live in the exotic islands of the Pacific eat a variety of fish, fruits, and vegetables. Herdsmen in parts of Europe and Russia drink low-fat cul-

TABLE 16   Low-Fat Protein Foods
(in Servings Providing 10 Grams of Protein)

Food	Amount	Grams Fat
Skim milk	9 oz.	0.1
Uncreamed cottage cheese	2 oz.	0.17
Cooked shrimp	1½ oz.	0.5
Cooked rice and beans	½ cup	0.7
Chicken (no skin)	1½ oz.	1.5
Pink salmon (canned)	1¾ oz.	3
Haddock	1¾ oz.	3.3
Veal (trimmed)	1½ oz.	4.5
Low-fat yogurt	10 oz.	5.0
Hamburger (lean)	1½ oz.	5.0
Hamburger (regular)	1½ oz.	8.5
Eggs (large)	1½ oz.	10.0
Ham	1½ oz.	10.0
American cheese	1½ oz.	13.5

tured milk, and eat whole-grain breads with fresh fruits and vegetables.

Compare the total fat and total fiber contained in the following two days' menus and get hints from them. Table 17 will help you select some of your favorite foods so that you can modify your diet to be higher in fiber.

Single Nutrients to Prevent Cancer

There are a number of claims that large doses of certain vitamins or minerals will protect against cancer. Some of these claims are based on theoretical considerations with little or no data to back them up. Others do not even have a theoretical reason for being used. And yet the practice of taking vitamin C or E or the mineral selenium to prevent cancer has become widespread. What little data we have in human populations do not show any protective effect for vitamin C. While high doses of vitamin C have not shown serious toxic effects, there has not been enough

High- and Low-Fiber Menus

Low-Fiber/High-Fat	*High-Fiber/Low-Fat*

Breakfast

instant orange drink	1 orange
1 slice white bread	1 slice whole wheat bread
1 tsp. butter	1 tbsp. apple butter
6 oz. whole milk	1 cup 40% bran flakes
½ cup canned peaches	6 oz. skim milk
1 cup cornflakes	1 tbsp. almonds and 1 tbsp. raisins

Lunch

3 oz. roast beef	3 oz. turkey (white meat) on whole wheat bread
1½ tbsps. mayonnaise	mustard and lettuce
20 french fries	tossed salad with lemon juice
6 oz. instant onion soup	1 cup vegetable soup
cola	8 oz. apricot nectar
gelatin dessert and topping	1 medium apple

Snack

snack pie	½ cup dried fruit-and-nut mix
coffee and cream	6 oz. vegetable juice

Dinner

4 oz. fried chicken	4 oz. broiled fish
½ cup macaroni and cheese	1 cup gumbo (corn, tomatoes, okra)
¼ cup cole slaw	1 cup brown rice
½ cup buttered peas	1 cup fresh relish (radishes, celery, green pepper, carrot curls)
2 dinner rolls	1 slice Banana Bran Bread (see recipe)*
2 tsps. butter	¼ canteloupe wedge
¾ cup ice cream	

High- and Low-Fiber Menus

Low-Fiber/High-Fat   High-Fiber/Low-Fat

Snack

10 potato chips   1½ cups popcorn (plain)
12 oz. carbonated beverage   12 oz. apple juice

Total

127 grams fat   45 grams fat
4.7 grams fiber   17.23 grams fiber

*Banana Bran Bread

½ cup butter or margarine   1½ cups unsifted all-purpose
¾ cup sugar   flour
2 eggs   2 tsps. baking powder
1½ cups mashed ripe   ½ tsp. baking soda
  bananas   ½ tsp. salt
1 tsp. vanilla
1 cup bran

—mix in large bowl: margarine, sugar, eggs, bananas, and vanilla.
—add bran and let stand for five minutes.
—mix dry ingredients together and blend with banana mixture.
—bake in greased, floured, 9 × 5 × 3″ loaf pan at 350°, 1 hour 10
  minutes.
—when done, cool for 10 minutes, then remove from pan, and
  cool on rack.

TABLE 17   Fiber Content of Some Common
            Foods

Food	Amount (Measure)	Fiber (g)
Almonds	½ cup	1.8
Apple, unpeeled	1 medium	1.5
Asparagus pieces, cooked	½ cup	0.3
Bananas	1 medium	0.9
Beans, green, cooked	½ cup	0.6

Food	Amount (Measure)	Fiber (g)
Bran, wheat	2 tsps.	1.0–2.0
Bread, white or French	2 slices	0.1
Bread, whole wheat	2 slices	0.9
Broccoli, chopped cooked	½ cup	1.2
Bulgur wheat, cooked	½ cup	0.5
Cabbage, cooked	½ cup	0.6
Cabbage, raw, shredded	½ cup	0.3
Carrots, cooked	½ cup	0.7
Carrots, raw	1 medium	0.5
Celery	1 stalk	0.3
Cornflakes	1 cup	0.2
Corn on cob, cooked	1 ear	1.0
Cucumber	½ medium	0.8
Lettuce, iceberg	⅛ head	0.3
Lettuce, romaine	2 leaves	0.4
Macaroni, cooked	½ cup	0.1
Mushrooms	10 small	0.8
Noodles, cooked	½ cup	0.1
Oatmeal, cooked	½ cup	0.2
Orange	1 medium	0.9
Orange juice	½ cup	0.1
Peanuts, roasted	½ cup	1.7
Peas, cooked	½ cup	0.5
Popcorn	3 oz.	2.0
Potatoes, baked in skin	1 medium	0.6
Potatoes, mashed	½ cup	0.4
Rice, brown, cooked	½ cup	0.3
Rice, white, cooked	½ cup	0.1
Soybeans, cooked	½ cup	1.0
Spinach, cooked	½ cup	0.5
Squash, summer, cooked	½ cup	0.6
Squash, winter, cooked	½ cup	1.4
Strawberries, raw	½ cup	1.0
Tomato	1 medium	0.8
Walnuts	½ cup	1.1

experience with these doses for long enough periods of time (over many years) to be sure. Vitamin E has been shown to offer some protection against certain cancers in animals. No studies in humans have confirmed this effect. High doses of selenium have not been shown to be effective against cancer in humans. In addition, there has been no experience with long-term administration of high doses of selenium, and there is reason to believe such a practice may be dangerous.

Vitamin A given in high doses has been shown to have a protective effect against various types of cancers. Vitamin A is extremely toxic in high doses and therefore cannot be used as a preventive measure. However, recently the structure of vitamin A has been altered in the laboratory so that its toxicity has been reduced while its cancer-preventing properties have been preserved. Several such "analogs" of vitamin A are currently being tested in populations at very high risk for certain cancers, for example, people with bladder papillomas (a precancerous condition) or asbestos workers, who are at very high risk for lung cancer. These tests have not yet reached a stage where any definitive judgment can be made about their efficacy. It should be noted that even in the animal experiments, these analogs, like vitamin A itself, are effective only as preventive measures. They are *not* a cure for cancer.

The experimental data with vitamin A coupled with some human studies indicating that populations with a high incidence of vitamin A deficiency also have a relatively high incidence of certain cancers has led to recommendations by some scientists that an abundant amount of vitamin A from plant sources be included in our diet. In practice this means eating lots of carrots, squash, and other yellow vegetables. While this is no sure way of preventing cancer, it seems a reasonable step to take. Many Americans tend to consume too little vitamin A, and no toxicity occurs when the amount of dietary vitamin A from vegetable sources is increased.

A few animal studies have suggested that certain foods may offer some cancer protection. The substance or substances within such foods have not been identified. Some cruciferous vegetables, particularly Brussels sprouts, have shown this effect. Although it certainly is too early to recommend a diet loaded with Brussels sprouts, these studies should be followed carefully and the anticancer substance, if one exists, identified.

While this chapter has focused on prevention it must be mentioned that a number of substances, some of them found in foods, have been touted as cancer *cures*. In some cases these claims have been made by well-meaning people, in others, by out-and-out charlatans. In either case, this is a very serious problem. Cancer victims are forgoing proven methods of treatment to try Laetrile or some other so-called remedy, and this practice is costing lives that may have been saved while draining the victim's family of its hard-earned savings. There is no known nutrient that will cure cancer. In situations where one or more nutrients have been tried, they have failed. Of course, if you or someone you know has cancer, high doses of vitamin C or vitamin E may be used but *in addition to* not *in place of* other therapy that has been shown to have beneficial effects. Remember, many cancers can be cured if proper therapeutic measures are undertaken early.

Chapter 7

Anemia

Your bloodstream is truly the "river of life." It carries the oxygen from your lungs to every cell in your body for use in generating energy, and it also carries the carbon dioxide, released as each cell expends energy, back to the lungs for release into the air. It carries both the nutrients that must be used as fuel and as building blocks for the growth and repair of tissues, and the waste products of tissue metabolism to be excreted by the kidney. In addition, your blood is a reservoir of cells able to be transported rapidly anywhere in your body to fight infection either by carrying immune substances or by actually engulfing invading organisms.

To carry out these essential functions the blood has evolved into a very special tissue containing a number of constituent parts, each of which is highly adapted to its job. There are two types of cells in the bloodstream: red cells and white cells. The white cells protect against infection; the red cells carry the oxygen and carbon dioxide. The red cells give the blood its color, and disturbances that cause either quantitative or qualitative changes in these cells will produce a condition known as anemia.

To understand what anemia is we must understand what a red cell is and how it is manufactured within the body. A red cell, or erythrocyte, is a very special cell highly adapted for its job as a carrier of oxygen and carbon dioxide. In its mature form the cell circulates through the blood as a small sphere filled with a substance called hemoglobin. Hemoglobin is a complex molecule made of two kinds of subunits: heme, a small iron-containing ringlike structure, and globin, a large chainlike protein molecule. It is the hemoglobin within the red cell that carries both the oxygen and the carbon dioxide. The more hemoglobin, the more seats available on the oxygen-carrying train; the less hemoglobin, the fewer seats. When the amount of hemoglobin drops below a certain level, the person becomes anemic. Simply stated, anemia means having too little hemoglobin.

To carry out its functions most efficiently, the red cell sacrifices certain properties that are present in all other cells. During its development it loses its nucleus, the discrete area within all cells that is responsible for maintaining many of the cell's life processes. As a consequence of this loss, the red cell has a much shorter life than any other cells in the body. The life-span of the average red cell is 120 days. Thus, every day about 8 percent of your red cells die and must be replaced.

These cells are replaced in the bone marrow, where cells that contain nuclei are dividing rapidly and constantly increasing in number. Some of these cells will then undergo a maturation process during which they will synthesize hemoglobin, lose their nuclei, and become mature red cells, which then will be released into the bloodstream to replace the red cells that are being lost. In other words, the bone marrow is constantly producing new red cells and supplying them to the blood as they are needed.

If we keep in mind this picture of hemoglobin-containing red cells constantly being lost and replaced, it is easy to understand how anemia can develop. If red cells are lost faster than they can be replaced, the total amount of hemoglobin circulating in the blood will drop and you will become anemic. Such an imbalance between the rate of red-cell loss and the rate of replacement can occur either because the cells are being withdrawn from the bloodstream too rapidly or because they are released in the bone marrow too slowly.

Both of these situations can and do occur, and both may have important nutritional implications.

Perhaps the most obvious situation in which red cells and the hemoglobin they contain are lost from the body is when you bleed. When the bleeding is mild, the bone marrow is able to compensate by producing red cells faster and by rapidly releasing them into the bloodstream. This will prevent the hemoglobin levels from falling and anemia from occurring. When the bleeding is severe, even if the bone marrow is working at capacity, it is unable to replace the lost red cells quickly enough and anemia will ensue. Therefore, whether or not you will become anemic following blood loss depends on how well your bone marrow is able to supply new red cells, and this ability of your bone marrow to respond depends in part on the state of your nutrition.

As we have seen, new red cells are constantly being manufactured in the bone marrow. For this to occur smoothly, the immature red cells must divide rapidly and new hemoglobin must be synthesized within the maturing red cell without hindrance. Both of these processes depend in part on the availability of certain nutrients. Three nutrients that are absolutely essential for cell division are folic acid, vitamin B_{12}, and zinc. One nutrient is crucial in the synthesis of hemoglobin: iron. A deficiency in folic acid, vitamin B_{12}, or zinc will cause a reduced rate of cell division within the bone marrow and hence in the production of fewer red cells. The result is anemia. A deficiency of iron will result in a reduced synthesis of hemoglobin within the maturing red cell, and eventually anemia will develop. Thus, the most common forms of nutritional anemia are caused by inadequate supplies of iron, folic acid, vitamin B_{12}, and zinc to the bone marrow. The most important factor in determining these supplies is your diet.

Iron Deficiency

Iron is so important to the body that specific mechanisms have evolved for its conservation. Iron is an integral part of hemoglobin, and most of the iron in our bodies is present in this form. However, it is also present in small amounts in every other cell in the body as part of the enzyme systems necessary for cell respiration. Finally, iron is present in muscle cells in a molecule known as myoglobin, which is important in voluntary muscle function. Iron can also be stored in the liver, spleen, intestines, and to some extent in other organs. Almost all the iron released from cells, including that released by dying red cells, circulates in the blood to storage sites to be held for release when it is needed. Thus, under normal conditions when no blood is lost from the body, very little iron is lost; almost all is reutilized by the body. Even a blood loss caused by injury to the tissues, such as in a bruise, releases iron that the body can reutilize.

Dietary iron requirements for an adult male are small and iron deficiency in adult males is rare. When it occurs, it usually signals bleeding from an unseen site and this is therefore a serious symptom that requires immediate medical attention. By contrast, during the human growth period, iron deficiency is quite common in both sexes and is usually due to inadequate dietary intake of iron. During growth the volume of blood circulating through the body must grow proportionally. Hence, more red cells are constantly being added over and above those that are lost, more hemoglobin is being synthesized, and more iron is therefore required. For example, an infant's blood volume can double during the first year of life. The one-year-old has twice the number of total red cells as the newborn and, hence, twice as much body iron. If a good supply of dietary iron is not available, iron deficiency and possibly anemia will occur. Adolescence is another period of extremely rapid growth when the total number of circulating red cells must increase. It also is a period in which iron deficiency may develop.

The adult woman during her reproductive life is also at risk for iron deficiency, since she regularly loses blood through menstruation. Again, if her intake of dietary iron is inadequate to meet the demands imposed by this constant iron loss, she will develop an iron deficiency and, eventually, the anemia that accompanies this condition.

Anemia is the last stage of iron deficiency. It occurs only after the iron stores within the body have been exhausted. For this reason even a mild anemia due to iron deficiency should not be ignored. It means all your iron stores have been used up, and in addition you are not consuming enough iron to keep the levels of hemoglobin in your blood high enough for optimal body function.

Pregnancy is a period in a woman's reproductive life when she is particularly at risk for iron deficiency. Her own blood volume expands, hence more red cells must be manufactured to meet this expansion. In addition, the fetus is growing and developing rapidly. Part of that growth is the establishment and rapid expansion of its own blood supply. This requires iron, which must come from the mother—either from her diet or from her iron stores. Since the storage of iron is cumulative, the more pregnancies a woman has undergone, the greater her risk for iron deficiency both during subsequent pregnancies and between them. Pregnancy places such a demand on iron requirements that iron supplements are routinely prescribed for pregnant women in the United States.

Iron deficiency is a progressive condition beginning with a slow depletion of iron stores, proceeding to mild, then moderate, and finally severe anemia. The rate at which anemia develops depends partly on the existing level of iron stores and on the difference between the amount of iron lost and the amount present in the diet. Let us suppose you have iron stores of 1,000 mg, you consume 10 mg per day of usable iron, and you lose 15 mg per day (this includes menstrual losses prorated on a daily basis). You are losing 5 mg per day more than you are absorbing, and in 200 days your entire iron reserves will be used up and anemia will begin to develop. Even a loss of 1 mg per day more than your body absorbs will result in a depletion of your entire iron reserves in less than three years. If you give blood, have an accident that involves blood loss, or suffer a nosebleed, these must be factored into the equation. For a woman the key to preventing iron deficiency is to absorb more iron than she is using over the long term. We call this being in positive iron balance.

A variety of foods contain iron in large amounts; therefore, it is reasonable to ask why anyone should be in negative iron balance. There are two reasons. First, the body will absorb only a small fraction of the iron present in food. Exactly how much depends on a number of factors—the kind of food, the other components of the diet, and the state of your iron reserves. Second, the "modern" life-styles of many American women reduce the amount of iron available in their diets.

Iron Absorption

Iron is absorbed by an active process in the small intestines. First, it is changed by the hydrochloric acid in the stomach into a form that can be absorbed, and when it reaches the small intestine, it is carried into the surface cells by the protein ferratin. This protein binds the iron, pulls it into the intestinal cell, where it is either deposited as storage iron or released into the bloodstream for transport to distant storage sites or to bone marrow for immediate use. While in the bloodstream, the iron is transported bound to another carrier protein, transferrin, which circulates in the plasma. The amount of iron absorbed depends on the nature of the iron-containing food, the other components of your diet, and the state of your iron reserves.

Iron is present in our food supply in two forms: heme iron, which has been derived from hemoglobin, and nonheme iron. Heme iron is contained primarily in meat, fish, and egg yolks; nonheme iron is found in vegetables and plant sources in general. About 15 to 20 percent of the heme iron in your diet will be absorbed. By contrast, only about 5 percent of nonheme iron will be absorbed. In the usual mixed American diet only about 10 percent of dietary iron is absorbed. For any individual, however, the amount of absorption will vary. If you are a vegetarian, you will absorb less than 10 percent; if you eat a great deal of meat, more than 10 percent. Table 18 shows the iron content of a variety of food.

Regardless of the source of dietary iron, its absorption is influenced by other components of the diet. Vitamin C consumed at the same meal will increase iron absorption. Thus, the orange juice you drink at breakfast will increase the iron you absorb from eggs or fortified cereal. By contrast, certain components of cereal grains known as phytates interfere with iron absorption. This is not a problem in the usual American diet because our major grain sources—wheat, corn, and rice—are not rich in phytates and what phytate content they have is almost entirely removed in processing. In some countries, such as Egypt and other Middle Eastern countries, however, staple grains are high in phytates, and the absorption of iron as well as other minerals can be diminished.

Probably the most important factor determining how much iron you will absorb is the state of your iron reserves. When your reserves are low, absorption is high. When they are high, absorption is lower. In other words,

TABLE 18   Iron Content of Foods in Milligrams (mg)
      Per Serving

.3–.7mg/serving

Fruit: e.g., apples, bananas, cherries, melons, citrus, pineapple, etc.	avg. size
Corn grits	1 cup
Popcorn (popped)	1 cup
Bread (all varieties)	1 slice
Enriched macaroni, spaghetti or noodles	½ cup
Peanut butter	2 tbsp.
Mushrooms	⅓ cup
Eggplant	½ cup
Tomato	1 small

.7–1.4 mg/serving

Rice, cooked (brown or white enriched)	1 cup
Tortilla (6 in. diam.)	1
Cream of Wheat	1 cup
Wheatena	⅔ cup
Wheat germ	1 tbsp.
Dry bulgur wheat	2 tbsp.
Pumpkin seeds	1–2 tbsp.
Berries (all)	1 cup

Broccoli	1 cup
Carrots	1 cup
Collards	1 cup
Potato	1 med.

1.5–2 mg/serving

Barley	½ cup
Buckwheat	½ cup
Oatmeal	1 cup
Chicken (all cuts)	3–4 oz.
Bologna	3–4 oz.
Ham	2 oz.
Dried apricot halves	6 large
Green beans	1 cup
Brewers' yeast	1 tbsp.

2–4 mg/serving

Amaranth	3½ oz.
Figs, dried	3 med.
Cooked peas & beans	½ cup
Blackstrap molasses	1 tbsp.
Tofu (soybean curd)	4 oz.

4–5 mg/serving

Beef (lean only), all cuts	3 oz.
Lamb (lean only), all cuts	4 oz.
Calf's liver	1 oz.
Raisins	½ cup

the body regulates the amount of iron absorbed depending on how much is already present. Somehow a signal is sent to the cells lining the small intestine to hold back or speed up iron absorption. The nature of that signal, however, is not known. This internal regulating system for iron absorption is a very important protection against both deficiency and overload. When iron is abundantly available, the body will absorb only what it needs. Unfortunately, for a variety of reasons iron may not be abundantly available. If it is not, even with increased absorption the body cannot make up the deficit, and iron deficiency occurs.

Factors That Limit Availability of Iron

For you to get enough dietary iron for your needs, your food must contain sufficient amounts of it. Any diet that is low in calories will restrict your food intake, thereby limiting the amount of iron available. For example, a woman on a 1,200-calorie diet would have to eat liver twice a week to get her iron requirement. How many women would do this? Below 1,200 calories it becomes almost impossible for a woman to meet her iron requirement from food alone. Therefore, a woman who is constantly dieting is at increased risk for iron deficiency, and the lower her caloric intake, the greater that risk.

Consuming large amounts of alcohol will interfere with iron absorption. A woman who is a moderately heavy drinker and who limits her caloric intake is in double jeopardy. Since many American women routinely practice calorie control and consume moderate amounts of alcohol, iron deficiency is extremely common in this population.

Folic Acid Deficiency

The vitamin folic acid is essential for normal cell division. The more rapid the rate of cell division, the higher the requirement for folic acid. In the adult the constant replacement of red cells by rapidly dividing marrow cells makes the bone marrow a tissue where cells are dividing more rapidly than elsewhere in the body. Folic acid deficiency will therefore manifest itself primarily in the bone marrow by reducing the rate of cell division. When this rate is reduced sufficiently to compromise the marrow's ability to replace lost red cells, the number of red cells in the blood will fall and anemia will result. The faster the red cells have to be replaced, the greater the need for folic acid. Women replace their red cells quicker than men because they must constantly make up for the blood losses of menstruation. Although there is no direct evidence, it is logical to assume that a woman's requirement for folic acid may vary at different times during the menstrual cycle. Thus, women require more folic acid than men, and anemia due to folic acid deficiency is more common in adult women than in adult men. The heavier a woman's menstrual losses, the greater her need for folic acid.

Unlike iron, folic acid is not stored by the body in appreciable amounts; hence, adequate quantities must be consumed daily and the requirement will increase during periods of great demand for new red cells. Also unlike iron, almost all the folic acid in your diet is absorbed. The excess is simply excreted. As with iron, however, constant calorie control will limit the amount of folic acid available in your diet even more than it will limit the amount of iron because your body has no control over how much folic acid is absorbed and therefore cannot extract more of this nutrient from your food if your reserves are low. Thus, if you are anemic because of folic acid deficiency, your body cannot protect itself by absorbing a greater amount of this nutrient from your food. Folic acid deficiency is *the* most common vitamin deficiency in the United States (see Table 19 for foods rich in folic acid).

TABLE 19   Folic Acid Content of Foods in Micrograms (mcg) per Serving

5–20 mcg/serving		*20–50 mcg/serving*	
Carrot	1 med.	Green beans	1 cup
Ear of corn	1 med.	Cucumber	1 small
Mushrooms	3 large	Squash	⅔ cup
Potato	1 med.	Strawberries	1 cup
Apple	1 med.	Egg	1 large
Hard cheese	1 oz.	Kidney	3 oz.
Grapefruit	½ med.	Shellfish	6 oz.
Milk	8 oz.	Yogurt	8 oz.
Bread	1 slice		
Sesame seeds	1 tbsp.		
Lean beef, veal, or pork	6 oz.		
100–150 mcg/serving		*200–300 mcg/serving*	
Liver (all)	3 oz.	Brewers' yeast	1 tbsp.
Broccoli	2 stalks	Spinach	4 oz.
Orange juice	6 oz.		

Even a moderate consumption of alcohol will reduce the amount of folic acid you absorb and will therefore increase your risk for this deficiency. Certain drugs can also affect folic acid metabolism and result in a deficiency. Perhaps the most important drug in this respect is the contraceptive pill, which may both decrease absorption and increase excretion of folic acid. The result is that many women who use oral contraceptives are at increased risk for folic acid deficiency. This problem is often compounded by the fact that increasingly, women are planning their pregnancies and timing them carefully; therefore, they stop taking oral contraceptives so that they can become pregnant. If they succeed, and particularly if they succeed quickly, they may enter the early stages of pregnancy relatively deficient in folic acid. Because pregnancy is accompanied by rapid cell division in the developing fetus, and because both maternal and fetal bone marrow are very active in making new cells, a woman's folic acid requirement increases dramatically. A deficiency during early pregnancy may be associated with certain types of congenital malformations. If the deficiency occurs later in pregnancy, it may result in the mother's developing anemia. Therefore, it is currently recommended that every pregnant woman take folic acid supplements, particularly if she has been taking oral contraceptives for a long time prior to pregnancy. In this case she should begin the supplementation as soon as she discontinues taking the pill.

Other Nutrient Deficiencies

Zinc

The mineral zinc, like the vitamin folic acid, is necessary for cell division. Thus, the demand for zinc will increase when the bone marrow is very active and during pregnancy when cell division increases in both the mother and the fetus. Zinc is often found in the same foods as iron. Hence, people who are iron deficient are often also zinc deficient. Like iron, zinc is stored in the body, and there is some evidence that the state of your zinc reserves influences the rate at which your body absorbs this mineral from food. Unlike iron, zinc is not a structural element in hemoglobin or any other major blood protein. Blood loss is not accompanied by the loss of large quantities of zinc. However, the response of the bone marrow to blood loss increases the zinc requirement. Thus, women of childbearing age need increased zinc not because lost zinc has to be replaced, but rather because more red cells have to be made.

As with the other nutrients involved in nutritional anemias, zinc deficiency will result if the increased demand is not met adequately by the dietary supply. The amount in the diet is, in turn, limited by the quantity and quality of the food consumed and by the life-style of the individual. Again, limiting the number of calories means limiting the amount of food and results in an increased risk for zinc deficiency. If the diet is low in foods with a high zinc content, that risk is compounded. (See Table 20 for foods rich in zinc.) Alcohol reduces zinc absorption and therefore increases your risk for deficiency.

Even if your body is deficient in zinc, you are not likely

TABLE 20   Zinc Content of Foods in Milligrams (mg)
            per Serving

.2 to .5 mg/serving

Egg	1 med.
Gefilte fish	3½ oz.
Mango	½ med.
Applesauce	1 cup
Pineapple juice	8 oz.
Tomato	1 med.
Potato, cooked	1 med.

.5 to 1 mg/serving

Puffed wheat	1 oz.
Cheddar cheese	1 oz.
Tuna	3 oz.
White rice	1 cup
White bread	2 slices
Cranberry-apple drink	8 oz.
Chicken breast	3 oz.
Milk (whole or skim)	8 oz.

1 to 1.5 mg/serving

Clams	3 oz.
Brown rice	1 cup
Whole wheat bread	2 slices
Popcorn	2 cups
Wheat germ	1 tbsp.
Bran (cooked, dried)	¾ cup.

4 to 5 mg/serving

Beef (lean only)	3½ oz.
Pork (lean only)	3½ oz.
Lamb (lean only)	3½ oz.
Liver (beef and calf)	3 oz.

Other

9.4 mg—Pacific oysters (raw)	3½ oz.
74.7 mg—Atlantic oysters (raw)	3½ oz.

to become anemic. There are two reasons. First, it takes a greater degree of depletion to cause anemia from zinc deficiency than it does from an iron or a folic acid deficiency. A person with iron-deficiency anemia will often be zinc deficient as well (because the same foods tend to supply both nutrients). The anemia, however, will be caused by the lack of iron, not the lack of zinc, since even a moderate iron deficiency often rapidly results in anemia. Therefore, iron-deficiency anemia should be treated not *only* with iron supplements, since these do not usually contain zinc. By increasing your consumption of iron-rich foods, you will increase your zinc intake and, we hope, establish an eating pattern that will prevent subsequent deficiencies.

Secondly, even a relatively severe zinc deficiency will often manifest itself in other signs before anemia develops. These signs include skin problems, taste abnormalities, endocrine problems, and in children, growth and sexual maturation problems. It is important to remember therefore that even if you are not anemic because of a zinc deficiency, your zinc reserves may be low enough to cause other problems. This is particularly important for women of childbearing age because zinc deficiency has been associated with congenital malformations of the fetus. These malformations occur at low serum-zinc levels in the mother even if other signs of deficiency are absent. Because zinc deficiency is so prevalent in women who are iron deficient, I believe that any pregnant woman who is iron deficient should take iron and zinc supplements.

Vitamin B_{12}

One of the major manifestations of vitamin B_{12} deficiency is anemia. This type of anemia is identical to the anemia that results from folic acid deficiency because vitamin B_{12} is necessary for folic acid to work properly. In essence, a person who has a vitamin B_{12} deficiency also lacks folic acid not because the latter is missing in the diet, but because it cannot be properly used by the body. Vitamin B_{12} is found in all foods of animal origin and is required only in small amounts. Hence, with the exception of *pure* vegetarians, dietary vitamin B_{12} deficiency almost never occurs. Vitamin B_{12} is also the only water-soluble vitamin that is stored in the body. It takes about three years for a person's normal reserves to be depleted. Hence, anemia caused by a vitamin B_{12} deficiency takes a long time to develop, and unless there is some abnormality (such as the body's inability to absorb the vitamin), the condition should occur only in pure vegetarians. Nutritional anemia resulting from a diet deficient in vitamin B_{12} is very rare.

Other Nutrients
Anemia can occur because of a lack of other nutrients in the diet but it is extremely rare. Nutrient deficiencies that have been implicated in anemia are copper and vitamin E. However, the deficiencies must be prolonged and severe before anemia results; therefore, only people with extremely unorthodox eating habits are at risk from a lack of copper and vitamin E in their diets.

Anemia Resulting from Combined Nutrient Deficiencies

Since the conditions necessary for the development of iron-deficiency anemia and folic-acid-deficiency anemia are often similar, some women can become anemic because they lack both nutrients. It is extremely important to diagnose such a condition. Treatment with iron or folic acid alone will not cure this anemia. Fortunately, your physician will be able to tell if you have a combined anemia by examining a drop of your blood. As we shall see, this is only one of many reasons why self-treatment of anemia is not advisable. Treatment of a combined anemia is simple— supplementation with both iron and folic acid. Prevention of a recurrence may involve a change in life-style and will certainly involve a change in diet.

Anemia that results from a combination of other nutrient deficiencies is quite rare. Occasionally a woman who is a pure vegetarian (vegan) may develop an anemia caused by a lack of both iron and vitamin B_{12} in her diet. This happens because the best source of iron is meat and other animal products, and vitamin B_{12} is found *only* in animals and animal products. However, even small amounts of meat, fish, or dairy foods will supply your vitamin B_{12} requirement. Therefore, the vegan who is anemic is most likely iron deficient, and only rarely deficient in vitamin B_{12}.

Signs and Symptoms of Nutritional Anemias

Regardless of the cause of the nutritional anemia, the general signs and symptoms are the same because they result from the same abnormality, too little hemoglobin in the blood. Hemoglobin is red in color, which is reflected in the body, particularly where the blood comes close to the surface, such as the nail beds, the tips of the fingers and toes, the earlobes, and the skin around the eyes. Anyone who is anemic will display a lightening in color in these areas—usually ranging from pink to a grayish-white. This will occur no matter what the pigmentation of your skin and can be recognized by a trained eye. As the anemia progresses, a general pallor will develop and this too will be noticeable no matter what color your skin is. One way to test for anemia is to press on your nail beds until they become white, then release the pressure—a prompt return to pink is the normal response. If the pink returns very slowly, then anemia must be suspected.

Hemoglobin carries oxygen from the lungs to the tissues. If not enough hemoglobin is present, not enough oxygen is reaching the tissues and certain signs and symptoms will develop because of this lack. Tiredness and general fatigue are among the earliest signs. Your attention span becomes shorter and you begin to do poorly at your job, particularly if you work at something that requires concentration. You become listless and irritable. You lose patience and the least bit of exertion bothers you. Finally, you can become weak and short of breath. All these symptoms are nonspecific; that is, they can occur with conditions other than anemia. Therefore, your physician will examine your blood. A low hemoglobin value signifies anemia.

Once anemia has been diagnosed, its cause must be established. Anemia may result from a number of causes other than faulty nutrition. In some cases it may be a sign of a very serious disease. Therefore, it is essential that the cause of that anemia be found. For example, certain diseases of the blood or bone marrow will produce anemia. The marrow may "break down" and not be able to replace the red cells that are constantly being lost. No kind of nutritional treatment will cure this kind of anemia. Sometimes the red cells themselves break down much more rapidly than normal. This condition may be due to genetic abnormalities in the red cells, as in sickle-cell anemia, or to ingestion of or exposure to certain toxins that cause red cell damage.

Perhaps the most common nonnutritional cause of anemia is bleeding. The blood loss may be slow and not easily recognized; for example, bleeding from the gastrointestinal tract. Unlike the anemias mentioned above, that caused by bleeding *will* respond to nutritional treatment. Iron is being lost and the anemic condition is due to iron deficiency—not because of insufficient iron in your diet, but rather because you are abnormally draining your iron stores. Iron supplementation will cure the anemia but not the disease—a very important principle to remember.

If it is iron-deficiency anemia, why are you iron deficient? In women it is usually because their iron intake is not sufficient to meet their bodies' normal demands, or because of heavy menstrual periods or one or more pregnancies that may have drained their iron reserves. They may consume a diet that does not supply enough iron. In men, however, iron deficiency rarely occurs because of too little iron in the diet, since an adult male's normal requirement is very small. Iron-deficiency anemia in an adult male must be considered a sign of abnormal bleeding until proven otherwise, and the cause of the bleeding must be established. Self-treatment with iron may temporarily correct the symptoms of iron deficiency, but you are actually delaying the diagnosis of the actual problem and you may seriously jeopardize your health.

Anyone who is anemic should see a physician to determine the cause. In a woman who has no other physical problems if the condition is due to iron deficiency the physician may decide to use an iron supplement and recommend a diet high in iron. In a man a much more extensive series of diagnostic tests must be undertaken to determine the cause of iron loss. Only if no source of bleeding is found will iron supplementation be undertaken.

Who Is at Risk?

The populations mainly at risk for nutritional anemias are women during the childbearing years and children of both sexes during their growing years. In addition, there is some evidence that certain elderly men and women may be at increased risk. Unlike the case of most of the other diseases we have discussed, your race or family history is not important in determining your risk. There are no known genetic factors that increase a person's chances of developing nutritional anemias. Similarly, other factors such as smoking, high blood pressure, obesity, and lack of exercise—so important in many of the diseases already discussed—do not influence your risk for developing a nutritionally induced anemia. However, for the population groups mentioned above there are certain other risk factors that can increase their chances of developing nutritional anemia.

Women During the Childbearing Years

During the childbearing years, women go through certain cyclic changes in their physiology that put them at increased risk for developing nutritional anemias. Primary among these physiologic states are menstruation, pregnancy, and lactation, each requiring specific nutrients. In addition, during this childbearing period, many women have established certain life-style practices that increase their risk for nutritional anemias. The use of the contraceptive pill increases the need for folic acid; certain types of diets reduce the availability of iron, zinc, and folic acid. Excess use of alcohol reduces the absorption of the same three nutrients. This combination of life cycle and life-styles places the adult American woman at greater risk for nutritional anemias than the adult man. The extent of that risk depends on how these factors interact in each individual. It is important for any woman to establish her own risk for developing anemia, which can be done more precisely with this condition than with any of the diseases we have discussed.

Menstruation

How heavy are your menstrual periods? This is perhaps the most important question you have to answer in establishing your risk for developing nutritional anemia. Some women have very light menstrual periods and, as a result, lose relatively small amounts of iron; they require only small increases in dietary zinc and folic acid to replace the lost red cells. Other women lose copious amounts of blood with each period and must constantly struggle to renew their iron reserves, and to supply their bone marrow with enough zinc and folic acid to keep their bodies running at maximum efficiency. Most women fall somewhere in between. Try to determine the amount of blood you lose during an average period. First, how long does your period last? Three days, four, five, or more? Second, how many sanitary napkins do you use during each day of your period? Finally, is the amount of blood you lose every month predictable? In other words, are your periods similar in duration and extent each month, or do they vary considerably from month to month? In the latter case, it is much more difficult to determine your risk score. As we will see in the next section, it is better to err on the side of safety and use your heaviest periods as the criterion for determining your score.

Pregnancy

During pregnancy, of course, menstruation stops. However, the need for your own blood volume to expand and for the fetus to establish its own new blood supply more than balance this temporary stage without monthly blood loss. Your bone marrow works much faster during pregnancy; therefore, zinc and folic acid deficiencies are more common at this time. Hundreds of thousands of new red cells are pouring into your bloodstream from your own bone marrow and into the circulation of the fetus from its bone marrow. Each of these cells contains hemoglobin and therefore iron. All the iron must come from the mother—from her reserves, from her diet, or from both. During pregnancy a woman is more prone to develop anemia than when she is between pregnancies. Equally important, however, is that pregnancy can drain your reserves of iron and place you at greater risk for anemia afterward. The more pregnancies you have undergone, the greater your risk for nutritional anemia, particularly if you did not take iron and folic acid supplements during those pregnancies. If you have had twins or triplets, your risk is increased both during and after pregnancy. At delivery considerable blood can be lost. For this reason your physician will determine your hemoglobin and red-blood-cell count shortly after the baby is born. If these values are low, you will probably be given an iron supplement. However, even if they are normal, your nutrient supplies still may have been drained. Remember, anemia is the *last* stage of iron deficiency. It occurs only after all your iron stores have been depleted. In summation then, after pregnancy, your risk for nutritional anemia is increased, and the more pregnancies you undergo, the greater the risk.

Lactation

Nursing your baby will not increase your risk for nutritional anemia to anywhere near the extent that menstruation or pregnancy does. Your requirements for iron, zinc, and folic acid will increase, but so will your appetite. The increased food you will consume should go a long way toward helping you get enough of these nutrients. In fact, nursing women often do not resume menstruating until after the infant is weaned. Blood loss will be minimal; therefore, the nursing period is a good time to replace some of the nutrient stores depleted during pregnancy.

Oral Contraceptives

Although oral contraceptives have been shown to decrease the absorption of a number of vitamins, including folic acid and vitamin B_{12}, these drugs alone will rarely produce nutritional anemia. However, if a woman is already at high risk, using oral contraceptives may result in the anemia of folic acid deficiency. For some women, on the other hand, oral contraceptives reduce the severity of menstrual periods, in which case the risk for anemia is actually reduced.

Restricting Calories

Perhaps the greatest life-style factor influencing your risk for nutritional anemia is the reducing diet. As you lower your calorie intake more and more, you decrease your chances for getting your daily requirement of iron, zinc, and folic acid. Below 1,000 calories per day it is almost impossible for a woman to get her iron requirement from food alone. If you are continually dieting, your risk for developing anemia is increased. This is particularly true if the reducing diet is unbalanced. Remember, meat is the best source of iron and zinc, and certain vegetables are the best source of folic acid.

Vegetarianism

Increasing numbers of American women are practicing some form of vegetarianism. A potential problem in this practice is the increased risk of iron-deficiency anemia. Since meat is the best source of iron, and red meat in particular, a woman who eats little or no meat obviously is at increased risk for iron deficiency. She should construct her diet so as to provide a maximum source of vegetable iron. If eggs are part of her diet, the yolks are an excellent source of iron.

Alcohol

Alcohol consumed in even moderate amounts can increase your risk for nutritional anemia. It does so in two ways. First, it provides calories that are totally devoid of all other nutrients, thus cutting down the total number of nutrient-carrying calories you can consume. For example, suppose you are limiting yourself to 2,000 calories. If your diet is varied, you should be able to obtain your daily requirement of iron, zinc, and folic acid without much difficulty. But if you consume 500 calories from alcohol (less than five ounces per day), this leaves only 1,500 calories' worth of food to provide your entire daily requirement. This is much more difficult to achieve. Second, alcohol directly impairs the absorption of iron, zinc, and folic acid. This means the amount your body actually gets from your food is reduced; there is less food to supply the nutrients, and poorer absorption from what food you do consume.

Alcohol, even taken in moderate amounts, must therefore be weighed as a risk factor for nutritional anemia.

Both Sexes During the Growing Period

As your body grows, so does the volume of your blood, and the faster you grow, the more your blood volume expands. To keep pace with the expanding blood volume, the bone marrow must supply red cells faster. More zinc and folic acid are required. For these new red cells to mature and enter the bloodstream, more iron is required. Thus, during any period of rapid growth the risk for anemia increases. During fetal life the infant is rarely anemic, since the mother is supplying the nutrients required for the formation of fetal blood. However, the first year of life is a period of special risk. This is particularly true if the fetus is born prematurely. For the first few months of life the infant will consume breast milk or infant formula as its sole source of nutrition. Breast milk contains iron in a highly absorbable form, and if the mother's diet is well-balanced, folic acid is abundantly present in her breast milk. Zinc is also found in sufficient amounts in human breast milk. Thus, the breast-fed infant will rarely develop nutritional anemia. If the baby is bottle-fed, an infant formula that simulates breast milk and is fortified with iron should be used. When the infant is four months of age, solid foods may be introduced. However, breast milk or infant formula should still be used until the infant is nearly one year of age. Solid foods should emphasize the nutrients needed to prevent nutritional anemia, with the emphasis on iron. Many infant cereals are fortified with iron. Meat products and some strained green vegetables are also rich in iron. However, if the infant is a girl, preventing anemia is not enough. It is important also to ensure that her iron reserves are adequate. Unless this is done, she will start out in life with a disadvantage. When she needs to call on her iron reserves later in life, they will not be there.

The preschool years and the early school years are periods when growth proceeds at a moderate rate. Therefore, iron, zinc, and folic acid requirements will be somewhat increased. But these years are also a time of major physical activity and hence increased food intake. Rarely is supplementation necessary at this time unless the child is not receiving adequate amounts of a varied diet. If the family is strictly vegetarian, then the child could be iron deficient and fortified foods or an iron supplement may be warranted.

Adolescence is also a time of rapid growth, and nutritional anemias are common in both sexes. Because of their increased growth rate, adolescent boys develop anemia even more frequently than girls. However, from the standpoint of susceptibility to nutritional anemias in later life, the problem is more *serious* in girls. The adolescent girl with a nutritional anemia enters adulthood having exhausted her nutrient reserves, particularly those of iron, and hence her body is unable to meet the increased demands of menstruation and, later, of pregnancy. By contrast, the adolescent boy who is anemic will be able to make up the deficit much more easily as he stops growing and his body's demand for iron, zinc, and folic acid drops. Therefore, *during* adolescence both sexes have the potential for developing nutritional anemias, and children of either sex who are at risk, because of their very rapid growth coupled with a diet marginal in iron, zinc, or folic acid, should take preventive precautions. This is particularly true if they have any of the risk factors discussed earlier for the adult woman. For example, the adolescent who is constantly dieting is at increased risk, the vegetarian adolescent is at increased risk, and the adolescent who drinks alcohol to excess is also at increased risk. Particularly at risk is the adolescent girl who becomes pregnant. She herself is growing, her blood volume is expanding because she is pregnant, and her fetus is manufacturing new blood. The nutrients necessary to meet these demands may not be available even if her diet is good. Therefore, any adolescent who is pregnant should receive supplements of iron, zinc, and folic acid.

The Elderly

There is some evidence that older men and women may be more prone to nutritional anemias than young adults. The reasons are not entirely clear. Iron must be converted into its proper form for digestion by the hydrochloric acid in the stomach. Older people have less stomach acidity, and hence proper conversion may not take place. Thus, the amount of iron they take in with their food may be absorbed insufficiently to meet their needs. The stomach also produces a protein called intrinsic factor, which is necessary for the absorption of vitamin B_{12}. Again, in older people there is evidence that the production of this protein is reduced. Thus, over time an older person, particularly one who does not eat much meat or meat products, may develop anemia due to vitamin B_{12} deficiency. The evidence for folic acid deficiency is inconclusive. Some studies show that a high proportion of older people are deficient in this vitamin, others do not. Perhaps the biggest problem with determining whether aging is a factor in nutritional anemias is that many older people suffer from chronic diseases of all sorts. Some of these diseases may themselves increase the possibilities for developing anemia. Thus, in any older person anemia per se may be due not to dietary factors but to an accompanying disease. It is therefore important for any elderly individual who is even mildly anemic to see a physician to have the cause of that anemia determined.

Developing Your Personal Risk Score

Children and Adolescents
Both sexes are equally at risk for nutritional anemias during childhood and adolescence. A score of 5 or above places your child at high risk.

Infants

- Birth weight. Infants who weighed five and a half pounds or less at birth are at increased risk for nutritional anemias. Score 3 if your child falls into this category.
- Specific problems at birth. Any infant who has had an "Rh problem" or any other condition necessitating blood transfusions is at very high risk—score 5.
- Very rapid growth during the first year of life. If birth weight has more than doubled at four months or more than tripled at ten months, score 2.
- Bleeding during childhood. Severe nosebleeds, blood loss due to lacerations, and major surgical operations all increase risk. Score 2 for each.
- An infant formula that does not contain iron as the sole or major form of nutrition—score 3.

Any infant whose birth weight was low and who is growing rapidly would automatically be at high risk. Any infant who was of low birth weight and who suffers an episode of bleeding would be at high risk. Even an infant whose birth weight was adequate but who is growing very rapidly and being fed a formula that contained no iron would also be at high risk.

Since you do not know ahead of time whether your infant will grow rapidly or have nosebleeds or experience other forms of blood loss, it would be prudent to take certain precautions to prevent nutritional anemias in your infant. These precautions are simple: Breast-feed your child if you can. If you cannot or will not breast-feed, use an infant formula that contains iron. When you introduce solid foods (at around four months), choose those that are rich in iron, folic acid, and zinc.

Adolescence

- If you were at risk as a child (see above) and did not take preventive measures, your risk as an adolescent increases—score 3.

- If your growth rate is extremely rapid (more than three inches during any year), your risk increases—score 3.

- If you have had any episodes of significant bleeding before or during adolescence, your risk is higher—score 2 to 4 (depending on the severity of the bleeding).

- If you are a vegetarian, your risk is increased—score 2.

- If you begin your menstrual periods early (before age twelve)—score 3.

- If you are on a reducing diet—score 3. If your diet is unbalanced and low in iron, zinc, or folic acid—add 2 more points.

- If you are a "regular" user of alcohol—score 2; if you are a heavy drinker—score 3.

- If you become pregnant—score 5.

Thus, a person who was at risk as a child, and who undergoes very rapid adolescent growth, is at high enough risk to take preventive measures without any of the other factors being present. A rapidly growing adolescent who becomes a strict vegetarian or decides to go on a reducing diet is also at high risk and should take steps to prevent nutritional anemias. Of course, any adolescent who

For Adolescents of Both Sexes and Adult Women
(A score of 5 or more indicates high risk for anemia)

Risk Factor	Maximum Score	Your Score
History of Previous Risk	3	
Rapid growth	3	
Heavy menstruation	3	
Prolonged menstruation	2–3	
Previous pregnancies	1 (each)	
Twin pregnancies	2 (each)	
Bleeding at delivery	3	
Other significant bleeding	3	
Reducing diets	3	
Vegetarian (vegan) diet	2	
Use of contraceptives	2	
Consumption of alcohol	3	
Total	30 +	

becomes pregnant is immediately at high risk and should actually be taking iron, zinc, and folic acid supplements.

Women During the Childbearing Years

A score of 5 or more places you in the high-risk category.

- A history of high risk during infancy and/or adolescence—score 3.
- Heavy menstrual periods—score 3.
- Menstrual periods remaining heavy for more than three days—score 2. Lasting more than four days—score 3.
- Previous pregnancies (including miscarriages and induced abortions)—score 1 for each. Score 2 for each pregnancy resulting in twins.
- Bleeding complications at delivery—score 2.
- Other significant bleeding episodes—score 3.
- Frequent dieting to control weight—score 3.
- A pure vegetarian (vegan) diet—score 2.

- Use of oral contraceptives—score 2.
- Regular frequent consumption of alcohol—score 2. Heavy alcohol consumption—score 3.

As you can see, your previous history is very important. If you were at risk as a child or adolescent and did not take preventive measures, any of the other factors mentioned above automatically puts you into a high-risk category.

Diet for Those at High Risk

There are two main principles in constructing a diet that will protect against the development of nutritional anemias. First, the foods it contains must be of high nutrient density for iron, zinc, and folic acid. What I mean by high nutrient density is that the quantity of these nutrients *per calorie* in the daily diet should be as great as possible. Thus, a low-calorie food that is only moderately high in iron may be better than a high-calorie food that is very high in iron. Second, certain foods are extremely rich in these nutrients either naturally or because they are fortified. Some emphasis should be put on incorporating some of these foods into your regular diet.

To achieve the first objective, you need not only to eat certain foods but also to eliminate or at least markedly reduce others. Any food that supplies calories without these nutrients should be reduced. For example, alcohol and refined sugar have *no* nutrients, only calories. Therefore, a moderate reduction in these two "foods" can allow you to eat more nutrient-dense food without increasing your caloric intake. Fat, while carrying certain vitamins and supplying essential fatty acids, does not contain any of the nutrients that are important in protecting you against anemia. Hence your intake of fat, the most calorie-dense of all the nutrients (9 calories per gram), should be lowered substantially.

First, calculate roughly how many calories you are taking in (or wish to, if you are planning to lose weight). Then calculate how many calories you can eliminate by reducing alcohol, sugar, and fat consumption. Finally, decide what foods you will eat to increase your intake of iron, zinc, and folic acid to help protect against anemia. In some cases, as we will see, you will not be able to do this without eating fortified foods or taking supplements.

Nutrient Requirements for People at Risk

How much iron, zinc, and folic acid is necessary to prevent anemia? If you are not anemic yet, obviously you should take in more iron than you are losing and enough zinc and folic acid to allow your bone marrow to work at maximum efficiency. In the case of zinc and folic acid, supplying more than this amount will have little or no extra benefit. Therefore, any score over 5 would indicate that you should try to supply about one and a half to two times the recommended daily requirement. This amount should be more than adequate to meet your needs and allow your bone marrow to do its job. An adult woman's zinc requirement is 5 mg; hence, 10 mg per day is more than adequate. Similarly, 5 mg of folic acid (two times the adult female requirement) is adequate.

With iron, however, the situation is quite different. If you replace only the amount you are losing, you will avoid iron-deficiency anemia, but since your reserves are depleted, you will remain *at risk* for this anemia. To lower your risk you must rebuild iron stores. To do this you must take in considerably more iron than you are losing. How much more depends on how depleted you were initially. Your physician can determine this accurately, but it requires certain complicated tests. A less accurate but adequate method is to use your risk score to determine how much you must take in. The higher the score, the more depleted you are. A score between 5 and 10 should allow iron rebuilding with slightly more than the recommended daily requirement (18 mg), about 20 to 25 mg. For a person with a score between 10 and 20, 30 mg of iron daily would be reasonable. If your score is above 20, you should attempt to ingest 40 mg of iron per day. This last figure cannot be met from food alone unless you are consuming large numbers of calories and large quantities of iron-rich foods. A person with that high a score should be taking an iron supplement. Even taking 30 mg per day would be difficult for a woman, particularly if she is concerned about her calories. The use of iron-fortified foods is one option. If you choose a food containing 100 percent of the recommended daily allowance (RDA), 18 mg, then you need only 12 mg from the rest of your diet. Try to get that amount from meat sources—red meats (lean cuts) liver, and egg yolks—since that type of iron is better absorbed. If you do not wish to consume fortified foods, an iron supplement of 20 to 30 mg is indicated. If your score is between 5 and 10, you can get the iron you need from your diet if you choose foods carefully, avoid nutrient-poor foods, and consume adequate calories. If you are on a reducing diet, you should take an iron supplement. If you are a vegetarian and your score is 5 or above, you should take an iron supplement or eat iron-fortified foods.

The following simple chart may be useful.

Score	Requirement	Source
5–10	20–25 mg/day	diet, if calories are adequate
11–20	30 mg/day	diet plus fortified foods or supplement
21–30	40 mg/day	diet plus supplement

Planning a Diet to Prevent Anemia

First, decide how much iron you need using your risk score. Then decide if you need supplementation. If so, choose a supplement at an appropriate dosage (usually 20 to 30 mg per day). If you select fortified foods, pick one (usually a cereal) that contains 100 percent of the RDA for iron (18 mg); it may be fortified with zinc and folic acid as well.

Decide how many total calories you wish to take in each day (between 1,800 and 2,300 for the average woman; up to 2,800 for a very active woman). Decrease foods of low nutrient density (alcohol, refined sugar, fat). From Tables 18, 19, and 20 you can pick foods that are high in iron, zinc, and folic acid. Select generously to reach the amount you need. It may sound difficult to do, but it really isn't. Suppose you need about 25 mg per day of iron. You have the option of eating a fortified cereal several times per week, liver once a week, red meat twice a week, two to three eggs a week, spinach, collard greens, fish, raisins— all iron-rich foods. Choose the ones you like the best, but ensure your objective. And if the iron you need comes from your diet, you will also get enough zinc. An occasional seafood dinner, especially clams or oysters, will raise your zinc levels even more. Remember, iron and zinc are stored, so you need not get your exact requirement each day. You will want to average what you need over several days. A generous portion of oysters can supply a whole week's zinc requirement. One large portion of liver can supply your iron requirement for several days. In the case of folic acid, try to meet your requirement daily, since your body does not store this nutrient. This should be no problem if you eat a variety of foods listed in Table 17. Steps in planning a diet to prevent anemia are listed below:

- Set your requirement for iron, zinc, and folic acid.
- Decide on a supplement or fortified food.
- Decide on your total daily calorie intake.
- Decrease low-nutrient-density foods.
- Replace these with high-nutrient-density foods.

If you follow these simple steps, you can lower your risk for nutritional anemias by rebuilding your iron stores and keeping your bone marrow adequately supplied with zinc and folic acid.

Chapter 8

Osteoporosis

Every year more than half a million American women develop osteoporosis (brittle bones). Of these women, 200,000 over the age of forty-five will fracture one or more bones; 40,000 will die of complications following their injuries and thousands of others will be disabled, many seriously, for the rest of their lives. Osteoporosis and its complications is the twelfth most common cause of death in the United States, and in women it must be considered a major killer disease. And yet with all these impressive statistics, osteoporosis seems to be neglected. There are two possible reasons for this: One, brittle bones, are considered a natural result of the aging process; or two, until recently we have not been sufficiently concerned about the health of our older citizens.

How many times have we heard about a woman over sixty-five fracturing a hip and sorrowfully dismissed it as one of the inevitable consequences of getting older? Although osteoporosis is in a sense an exaggeration of the normal bone loss that accompanies aging in women, I hope in this chapter to dispel any notions that it is inevitable. Osteoporosis is a very serious and often debilitating disease and while it has no single cause, it is associated with a number of risk factors. Some of these risk factors are under your control; hence, your risk can be modified. Proper diet and certain kinds of exercise can reduce your risk. In this sense, osteoporosis is no different from atherosclerosis, hypertension, obesity, diabetes, and certain types of cancer. Like them, it is a disease that certain people are more prone to get than others. This chapter will try to explain what osteoporosis is, who is at risk, and how that risk may be minimized.

The Nature of Osteoporosis

Osteoporosis is simply a loss of bone. Therefore, to understand how it occurs it is important to understand the processes within our body that affect both bone growth and bone destruction.

Although bone is the strongest tissue in the body, it is not a solid mass. Bones are tubular structures with a central canal (marrow cavity) surrounded by a complex latticework of protein (collagen) and crystals made of calcium and phosphorus (hydroxyapatite). The marrow cavity is filled with blood-forming cells, which, though housed by bone, constitute a separate organ. In this cavity most of our blood cells are manufactured. From the marrow cavity these cells pass into the bloodstream by traversing millions of small blood vessels that must pass through the bone tissue itself. Thus, even bone tissue is not solid but is pierced by numerous blood vessels as well as by nerves. The blood vessels are not simply closed conduits passing from the circulation to the marrow, for in addition they nourish the bone tissue itself. Bone tissue, therefore, is in constant contact with the bloodstream, and through this contact the blood delivers substances to the bone and the bone releases substances into the blood. This intimate relationship between blood and bone is absolutely essential for the body to function properly. Bone is a living tissue and, as such, its protein matrix is constantly breaking down and rebuilding. As with all body proteins, bone collagen is in a state of perennial flux, moving new amino acids from the blood into its structure and releasing old amino acids from their products into the blood. In addition, however, bone is composed of a hard substance made mostly from the minerals calcium and phosphorus. This substance, called hydroxyapatite, is also constantly remodeling. Calcium and phosphorus move freely from the blood into the bone and from the bone into the blood. When new bone is being made, more calcium and phosphorus pass into the bone. When bone tissue is being destroyed, more of these minerals move out of the bone. If a similar amount is moving in and out of the bone tissue, there is no net change in bone mass.

Maintaining the structural integrity of bone is only one of the important functions of calcium. This mineral is essential for the proper working of every cell in the body. Without calcium, nerve cells cannot conduct impulses and muscle cells cannot contract. Calcium is essential for the brain to function and for the heart to beat. We cannot live unless calcium is available to all the tissues of the body. Ninety-nine percent of it is found in bone and only 1 percent circulates in our blood and is present in the other tissues. But this 1 percent is so critical that the body has evolved a complex machinery to keep the tissues supplied with just the right amount of calcium. This machinery is responsible for regulating the amount of calcium within the bloodstream, ensuring that the tissues get an adequate supply. At the same time, it protects them from receiving too much, for excess calcium within the tissues can have serious consequences. Bone plays a crucial role in this regulatory process.

The calcium in your bones is not only a major component of the mineral crystal that supports your body, but also a vast reservoir in which excess calcium can be safely stored and from which needed quantities can be withdrawn rapidly. If not enough calcium is available for your tissues, it will slowly be withdrawn from your bones. The more is withdrawn, the thinner your bones become. Eventually they become so thin that the everyday stresses of life are too much and fractures may occur. When your bones become like this, you are suffering from osteoporosis.

From the moment a calcium molecule enters your body from the food supply, the regulatory machinery in your body begins to act. First, the amount actually absorbed into your body is rigidly controlled by a hormone (dihydroxyvitamin D) made in the kidney from the vitamin D obtained from your diet or the vitamin D that has been activated by ultraviolet light in your skin. This hormone is necessary for calcium to be taken in by the intestinal cells and passed into the bloodstream. Once in the bloodstream, the calcium molecule becomes part of a whole population of these molecules, which represent the entire calcium level in the bloodstream. If this level should fall below a critical point, the parathyroid glands, four tiny glands at the base of the thyroid gland, secrete a hormone (parathyroid hormone). This hormone works to increase the level of calcium in your blood by signaling the kidney to convert vitamin D to its active form, thereby increasing calcium absorption, and by *stimulating the breakdown of bone,* which then will release its calcium into the bloodstream. To protect against too much calcium being withdrawn from the bones, the body uses another hormone, calcitonin, which is made in the thyroid gland. We do not understand yet how this hormone works, but somehow it inhibits the action of those cells within the bone tissues that break down the bone (osteoclasts). These three hormones, parathyroid hormone, dihydroxyvitamin D, and calcitonin, are the principal instruments employed in the body to regulate calcium metabolism. They are sensitive to the amount of calcium in the blood and they will react also to each other. In this way blood-calcium levels never get too high or too low.

Other hormones within your body play an important role

in determining whether bone loss will occur. These hormones are not involved in the regulation of blood calcium directly as are the three mentioned above. They are secreted for a variety of reasons, but not in response to the level of blood calcium. The most important is the female sex hormone estrogen.

Estrogen is a bone-protecting hormone. Yet it does not have any activity on bone itself. Estrogen works indirectly by blocking the action of parathyroid hormone. Thus when estrogen is present, greater amounts of parathyroid hormone are necessary to cause bone resorption and the release of calcium from bone to blood. If estrogen is not present, the brake is released, and even small amounts of parathyroid hormone will release large quantities of bone calcium. The fine tuning of the calcium-regulating mechanism is upset, more calcium gets into the blood than is needed, and the excess spills out into the urine, is excreted, and thereby lost to the body. In addition, estrogen stimulates the secretion of calcitonin (the primary bone-protecting hormone); so, when estrogen levels are low, calcitonin levels tend to be low and bone resorption tends to increase. Finally, recent evidence suggests that high levels of estrogen (like those occurring during pregnancy) stimulate the conversion of vitamin D to its active form in the kidney, thereby increasing the amounts of calcium absorbed and available for deposition into the bones. Thus, the absence of estrogen will produce an imbalance between the bone-resorbing hormone (parathyroid hormone) and the bone-protecting hormone (calcitonin), in favor of the former. As a result, calcium will be lost from the bones and excreted in the urine. In addition, the one hormone that might reverse this situation, dihydroxy-vitamin D, may not be made as efficiently in the absence of estrogen. Therefore, it is not surprising that menopause, when estrogen falls to very low levels, is the key event in the development of osteoporosis in women.

Another group of hormones affecting bone metabolism

TABLE 21

Bone Growth	*Bone Loss*
Primary	
Calcitonin	Parathyroid hormone
Dihydroxy-vitamin D	
Secondary	
Estrogen	Adrenocortical hormones
Progesterone	(Cortisone)
Growth hormone	Thyroid hormone

are the adrenocortical hormones. These hormones directly affect bone tissue, causing resorption. Both estrogen and another female sex hormone, progesterone, prevent the action of adrenal hormones on bone tissue. Thus, during menopause, when both of the sex hormones decline, the adrenal hormones are given greater license to cause a breakdown of bone. Finally, two other hormones affect bone. Growth hormone from the pituitary gland promotes growth of all tissues, including bone, while thryoid hormone promotes bone resorption.

Therefore, bone tissue is under a variety of hormonal influences within the body. Table 21 indicates those hormones which promote bone growth and those which promote bone loss.

When all these hormones are in balance, bone growth and loss are equalized and bone mass does not change. If the hormones that are involved in bone growth predominate (as they normally do during early life), bone mass will increase. If the hormones that are involved in bone loss predominate (as they normally do after menopause), bone mass will decrease. Anything that promotes the action or maximizes the effect of the bone-growth hormones will *lower* your risk for osteoporosis. Anything that promotes the activity or maximizes the effect of the bone-loss hormones will raise your risk for osteoporosis.

Now that we understand the relationship of the various

hormones to bone metabolism, let us trace the history of a typical bone as a woman goes through her normal life cycle. During infancy and early childhood, the bone-growth hormones predominate, and calcium is deposited into the growing bones. At puberty, estrogen and progesterone levels increase sharply, further promoting bone growth. During pregnancy, levels of estrogen and progesterone again rise, promoting bone growth in the mother and fetus. In addition, more dihydroxy-vitamin D is made during pregnancy by the placenta, which further promotes bone growth. If the mother nurses her infant, the levels of estrogen remain high and bone growth remains good. A few years prior to menopause, progesterone levels begin to fall and the balance tips in favor of the bone-loss hormones. At menopause estrogen levels fall dramatically and the bone-loss hormones become increasingly dominant. The result: bone is rapidly resorbed. At about age sixty-five, adrenal cortical activity lessens and levels of adrenal steroids like cortisone drop. This reduces the imbalance and bone loss slows down.

As we shall see, the best way to minimize your risk for osteoporosis is to take advantage of the periods when your hormonal balance favors bone growth. Unfortunately, most women wait to do this until they are near menopause or later when the balance of hormones is not in their favor. Under these circumstances, osteoporosis will often occur in spite of preventive measures taken. Thus, all women should do whatever possible during childhood and the childbearing years to promote maximum bone growth. Failure to do so among women who are at risk for this condition may result in severe and debilitating osteoporosis in their later years.

Besides internal forces, certain external forces will also influence bone growth and resorption. Primary are diet and exercise, particularly weight-bearing exercise. Obviously, no matter how efficiently your body deposits calcium into your bones, if you do not get enough of it in your diet you will not get enough into your bones. A diet deficient in calcium will promote bone loss. Not only is the amount of calcium in the diet important, but also how much can actually be absorbed from the gastrointestinal tract. Certain dietary elements promote calcium absorption and therefore promote bone growth indirectly. Other elements in the diet inhibit calcium absorption and therefore promote bone loss indirectly. We will examine these dietary interactions when we discuss eating practices that will lower your risk for osteoporosis.

Bones are made to bear weight, and weight bearing increases bone mass. When bones are not bearing weight, they lose mass. Thus, long periods of immobilization or bed rest will result in a loss of bone mass. The importance of weight bearing has become dramatically apparent in recent years through studies of astronauts. Even a relatively short period (two weeks) of weightlessness results in significant amounts of bone loss. In fact, this is the most significant medical problem facing our space program. Although research is currently under way, we still do not fully understand why the state of weightlessness induces such profound bone loss.

By now you must have guessed that osteoporosis is a disease more common in women than in men. This is because the main male sex hormone testosterone, like estrogen, is a bone-protecting hormone. Whether it works the same way as estrogen is still not known. However, since testosterone levels do not fluctuate in men the same way estrogen levels do in women, and since men do not undergo menopause, the overall balance between hormones that promote bone growth and those that promote bone loss remains better after they reach age forty-five or fifty. In addition, osteoporosis is a disease of older people. The older you are, the greater your risk for osteoporosis. Women live about eight years longer than men, and for that reason alone we can expect more women than men to become osteoporotic. Beyond these sex-hormone differences, males start life with a larger bone mass and naturally lose bone more slowly with age. They also have higher levels of calcitonin, and their increased weight and muscle mass place more stress on their bones.

Who Is at Risk?

Now that we understand what osteoporosis is and the major factors affecting bone resorption, we can determine who is at risk for this disease.

Your Sex
The first and most important general risk factor for osteoporosis is your sex. Women are ten times as likely to suffer from severe osteoporosis as men. However, men are not immune to the disease and as male life expectancy increases, more cases of osteoporosis will probably appear in them. As we shall see, many of the specific risk factors for osteoporosis will pertain only to women. Others, however, will pertain to both sexes. If you are male and have enough of these risk factors, it would be prudent to take preventive measures. The scoring system for osteoporosis risk, which is detailed in the next section, is constructed so that a woman is more likely to get a score that places her at risk than a man. However, some men will reach at least the lower levels of an at-risk score and these men should modify their diets just as women do who show high-risk scores.

Your Age at Menopause
The earlier you undergo menopause, the greater your risk for osteoporosis. Most women experience natural menopause between the ages of forty-five and fifty-five. Of these, about 25 percent will exhibit osteoporosis—with the percentage slightly higher below age fifty, and lower after age fifty. Women who have their ovaries removed prior to

natural menopause exhibit a 50 percent risk of developing osteoporosis. Again, the earlier the ovaries are removed, the greater the risk. Estrogen therapy may reduce the risk, but any woman who undergoes surgical removal of her ovaries before undergoing natural menopause must be considered at high risk.

Family History

Your family history is extremely important in determining your risk for osteoporosis. While the actual mechanisms by which your genes affect your bones are unknown, there is no doubt that a strong family history is an important risk factor. Try to fill in as many branches of your family health tree as possible. Remember, osteoporosis may not be an actual cause of death, so it is not enough just to ask what disease a relative died from. You must delve much deeper. Were there any fractures at older ages, particularly fractures of the hip or vertebrae? Did your grandmother limp? If so, at what age did she start? Was there a noticeable shortening of stature in any of your female relatives as they got older? If these symptoms appeared early or the relative involved is a close relation, the greater your risk for osteoporosis becomes. Taking a careful family history is important for men as well as women, since the genetic effect may be present in both sexes. Because osteoporosis is more prevalent in women, it may be your female relatives who will give you a clue to your own risk.

Your ethnic background must also be taken into account. Osteoporosis is less common among black women than among white women. Black women have larger bones at skeletal maturity. They also tend to have larger muscle masses that exert more stress on their bones. Black women also tend to lose bone naturally at a slower rate than white women, and some studies have shown that they also have higher blood levels of calcitonin. Thus, if you are a black woman you will be doubly protected. You start life with bigger bones and therefore can withstand more bone loss; you lose bone more slowly and hence will sustain less bone loss. Interestingly, there is no such protection afforded black men.

There have been only a few studies in other ethnic groups. Women whose ancestors came from the British Isles, northern Europe, China, or Japan are more likely to develop osteoporosis than those of African, Hispanic, or Mediterranean ancestry. The risk for Jewish women seems to fall somewhere between that of low-risk blacks and high-risk whites. Generally, there appears to be an association between actual skin pigmentation and the degree of risk. The whiter your skin, the higher your risk.

Body Build
If you are small in stature and narrow in build, your risk of osteoporosis is increased. You simply have less bone to start with, and given the same rate of loss, you will reach the osteoporotic, fracture-prone state more rapidly than your more sturdily built counterpart. This is true for men, too.

Body Weight
The thinner you are, the *higher* your risk for osteoporosis. Obese women rarely get the disease. The reasons are not entirely clear. We do know, however, that the more fat your body contains, the more estrogen it will be able to produce after menopause.

During a woman's reproductive life, the ovaries produce large quantities of estrogen and progesterone as well as small amounts of the male sex hormones androgens. The adrenal glands also produce androgens. After menopause the ovarian output of estrogen and progesterone drops to very low levels. However, the ovaries and adrenal glands still produce the same quantity of androgens. Fat tissue is able to convert these androgens to estrogens. The more fat tissue present, the more estrogen will be produced. Fat, therefore, reduces your risk for osteoporosis.

Another reason why very thin women (and men as well) have an increased risk for osteoporosis is that the amount of stress exerted on their bones is less than for heavier individuals and this results in increased bone loss.

Oral Contraceptives

Most oral contraceptives contain estrogen and progesterone, which stimulate bone growth. There is some evidence that women who take oral contraceptives, particularly if for a long time, may have greater bone mass when they enter menopause. Therefore, their risk may be somewhat less than that of women who have not used this form of contraception.

Number of Pregnancies

A woman who has never been pregnant has an increased risk for osteoporosis. During pregnancy, levels of estrogen and progesterone are very high and will promote bone growth provided calcium intake is adequate. Since increased estrogen levels will increase the production of the active vitamin D hormone made by the kidneys, and since the placenta will also make this hormone, calcium absorption is more efficient during pregnancy. With a diet adequate in calcium, pregnancy can be a period not only when your infant begins to form bone, but also a time for you to acquire stronger bones. Of course, if your diet is poor and your calcium intake low, the increased demand for calcium during pregnancy will be supplied by your bones, which will lead to a reduction of bone mass. This situation is frequently encountered in developing countries where women whose diets have been inadequate for most of their lives have repeated pregnancies.

Breast-Feeding

Although a large amount of calcium is "lost" each day if you breast-feed, there is no evidence that breast-feeding increases your risk for osteoporosis. In fact, there are theoretical reasons why the reverse may be true. Your hormonal milieu during lactation theoretically should promote bone growth. Much more research needs to be done on the relationship between lactation and osteoporosis, but currently the fear of osteoporosis is not a valid reason for not breast-feeding. In addition, breast milk will supply calcium to your infant in the most highly absorbable form available, and therefore give the newly forming bones a head start.

Exercise

If you have been confined to bed for a long period or have spent significant time in a wheelchair, you are at increased risk for osteoporosis. If you lead a sedentary life, your risk is higher than that of a person who is more active. Exercise that emphasizes weight bearing is important for several reasons. First, exercise places actual physical stress on your bones. Your bones respond by becoming bigger and stronger (hypertrophy). Second, exercise increases the flow of blood to your bones, thereby increasing the availability of bone-building nutrients. Third, exercise generates minielectrical currents within your bones that stimulate bone growth. Fourth, exercise alters your hormonal balance, favoring those that protect the bones. For example, one study indicated that middle-aged women had higher estrogen levels after a six-week period of moderate exercise. Another study found that middle-aged men who rode exercise bicycles had lower levels of the bone-resorbing adrenal hormones after they had exercised.

Actual measurements of bone density as a result of exercise have been done in a limited number of people. And these subjects, for the most part, were world-class athletes. To no one's surprise, the athletes had denser bones than the sedentary individuals who were used as controls. What is still unknown, however, is how much exercise is necessary to gain this increase in bone mass. Some studies suggest that regular exercise by middle-aged people over a sustained period of time (one year or more) will prevent the bone loss that would normally occur at this time of life. However, the number of subjects in these studies was small and more data are needed. At present, several long-term studies are under way to see if regular exercise can increase bone mass in various populations.

In summary, absence of exercise or leading an extremely sedentary existence will increase your risk for osteoporosis. Regular exercise may actually increase your bone mass and thereby reduce your risk or at least delay its onset.

It is important to note that the type of exercise that gives these results, such as walking, jogging, cycling, gymnastics, basketball, tennis, etc., tends to place a stress on your bones. Swimming, excellent for cardiovascular fitness, is a poor exercise for lowering your risk of osteoporosis. The buoyancy of the water takes the stress off your bones.

Smoking

If you smoke you are at greater risk for osteoporosis than if you do not smoke. However, it is still not clear whether smoking is an *independent* risk factor for osteoporosis. Women who smoke generally reach menopause about five years earlier than nonsmokers and, as we have seen, early menopause increases your risk for osteoporosis. Smoking is known to affect the function of the liver, which is involved in making the vitamin D hormone that increases calcium absorption, thereby protecting your bones. Smokers tend to be leaner than nonsmokers, and lean women are more at risk for osteoporosis. However, smoking per se may not increase your risk. Studies need to be done to determine exactly how smoking increases your risk. There is no reason, however, to await their results as there are plenty of other reasons for you to stop smoking right now.

Alcohol

Alcohol can have a profound effect on liver function and markedly reduce the production of the vitamin D hormone. Alcohol can directly impair the absorption of calcium through the gastrointestinal tract. Therefore, heavy consumption of alcohol can result in osteoporosis in both men and women at early ages. Men with alcoholism have exhibited severe osteoporosis in their twenties, probably because their livers are damaged, their diets are poor, and their exercise levels are low.

Currently we are not sure whether moderate consumption of alcohol over long periods of time will increase your risk for osteoporosis. However, if you are already at high risk, this may be just one more factor stacking the cards against you.

Medications

Cortisonelike Drugs

Among several chronic diseases that are treated over long periods of time with cortisone or derivatives of cortisone (hydrocortisone, prednisone, dexamethasone, etc.) are asthma, rheumatoid arthritis, and ulcerative colitis. These drugs can produce profound bone loss and result in severe osteoporosis in both sexes at early ages.

Cortisone and its derivatives appear to act in two ways: they increase calcium excretion and decrease calcium absorption, thus producing a net calcium loss. They also affect bone tissue, directly blocking the formation of new bone. While the osteoporosis induced by these drugs is quite similar to the form that occurs in postmenopausal women, the drug-induced disease is often more severe and often affects bones such as the ribs, which are generally spared in postmenopausal osteoporosis. However, the two diseases are additive; thus, anyone who has been treated with these drugs for a long time is at increased risk for osteoporosis.

Anticonvulsants

Drugs like phenytoin, phenobarbital, primidone, and phensuximide stimulate the production of enzymes in the liver that break down the vitamin D hormone produced by the liver. A relative vitamin D deficiency ensues and calcium absorption is impaired. The result is bone loss. Anyone taking these drugs is therefore at increased risk for osteoporosis.

Antacids

Millions of Americans use antacids regularly to alleviate the symptoms of everything from "acid indigestion" to peptic ulcer. Many antacids contain aluminum, which can cause an increase in the rate of calcium excretion. Sometimes antacids are used together with corticosteroids to prevent the gastric upset that these drugs often cause. Antacids are also frequently used by alcoholics. If you use antacids frequently, and particularly in the combinations outlined above, your risk for developing osteoporosis is increased.

Illness

Any illness that keeps you in bed for a long time will increase your risk for osteoporosis. In addition, certain specific illnesses will increase that risk over and above the effects produced by lack of weight bearing. Endocrine diseases, like hyperparathyroidism, hyperthyroidism, and overactive adrenals (Cushing's syndrome), will increase bone loss. Chronic diseases, such as diabetes, rheumatoid arthritis, and some forms of kidney disease, can also increase your risk for osteoporosis. Certain gastrointestinal problems, like sprue or celiac disease, will result in poor calcium absorption from your food and hence an increase in bone loss. If you have any of these diseases, your risk of osteoporosis is increased.

In addition, in some people periodontal disease may be similar to osteoporosis. Bone resorption takes place within the jawbones. Thus in some individuals periodontal disease may be a forewarning of osteoporosis to come.

Diet

A number of dietary factors can contribute to the development of osteoporosis. First, and most important, is a calcium deficiency. No matter how favorable your hormonal balance, if your diet is too low in calcium your bone mass will decrease. There are periods in life when a calcium deficiency is more dangerous than at other times, for example, the early growing years, particularly the infant years. At this time, bone is being produced at a rapid rate and hormonal balance is favoring bone growth. The reserves are already being built up for later life. If the diet is deficient in calcium at this time, or if calcium cannot be absorbed properly, the impaired bone growth that may result can never be replaced. Breast milk is the best food for a young infant, as the calcium it contains is better absorbed than calcium from cow's milk. For mothers who do not or cannot breast-feed, an infant formula that simulates breast milk as closely as possible is preferred for the greater part of the first year of life to ensure maximum calcium absorption.

Adolescence is another time when inadequate calcium intake can be very dangerous because it can lead to developing osteoporosis later in life. An adolescent undergoes the most rapid rate of bone growth that will occur during any period of his or her life. Unfortunately, many adolescents have eating habits that promote calcium deficiency. Some just eat foods that are low in calcium or high in phosphorus (which interferes with calcium absorption). Others diet so rigorously that they are not taking in enough food to supply their calcium needs.

Pregnancy is another period when insufficient intake of calcium can lead to a reduction of bone mass. The fetal skeleton is rapidly consuming calcium, and although the mother's body is in a hormonal state that favors bone growth, unless adequate calcium is available the maternal bones will be the only source of this mineral. If necessary, fetal bone growth will take place at the expense of maternal bone mass. A diet adequate in calcium will not only supply enough for your fetus, but also allow your own bones to increase their mass.

If you nurse your infant, your milk will have to supply large amounts of calcium, which is essentially lost to your body. If dietary calcium is inadequate during this period, again your bones must supply the calcium your milk lacks. Lactation is a critical time when a lack of dietary calcium can erode bones. Your body's hormones favor bone growth during lactation, and even with the calcium drain, you can finish nursing with an increase in bone mass if enough calcium is available to satisfy the needs of both your infant and your bones.

We have seen that the body regulates the amount of dietary calcium absorbed through the intestines into the blood as well as the amount excreted by the kidneys into the urine. This balance between absorption and excretion will determine whether sufficient calcium is available for bone growth or whether calcium must come from your bones to supply your tissues. Several other constituents in your diet will affect your calcium balance.

The first is vitamin D, which is so important that the body maintains two methods of getting enough. Your skin contains a substance which, when exposed to the ultraviolet rays of the sun, is converted to vitamin D. In addition, your food supply contains vitamin D naturally (in fish oils, for example) and through fortification (as in dairy products). However, vitamin D, whether consumed in the diet or converted from the skin, has very little activity within your body. To become an active compound it must undergo two chemical modifications. The first takes place in the liver, which manufactures an intermediate form of vitamin D between the form that occurs in nature and the final product made by the body. This intermediate form is somewhat more active than natural vitamin D, but is nowhere near as active as the final form, which is made in the kidney. This final form, sometimes called vitamin D hormone, is essential for calcium absorption. We have already seen how liver disease or kidney disease can interfere with the manufacture of this hormone and increase your risk for osteoporosis. However, even when your liver and kidneys are working perfectly, if not enough vitamin D is available for conversion to the active hormone, less hormone will be made. The results are poor calcium absorption, retarded bone growth, increased bone loss, and greater risk of osteoporosis. It is important, therefore, to get enough vitamin D. Too much, however, is of no advantage, since the body converts only as much as it needs. Also, too much vitamin D can be quite harmful, since it can result in the abnormal deposition of calcium in soft tissues such as the kidney.

The amount of phosphorus in your diet will also affect your calcium balance. Like calcium, phosphorus is a mineral that is essential for life. Also like calcium, the greatest amount of phosphorus is present in bone. Unlike calcium, however, phosphorus is present in such abundance in our food supply that primary phosphorus deficiency almost never occurs. In most American diets, there is such an excess of phosphorus that it can promote negative calcium balance. This happens because calcium and phosphorus are transported from the intestines into the blood by the same system. These minerals do not diffuse passively through the intestinal wall, but are actually borne by protein molecules specially adapted for this work. These "carrier" molecules have a specific and limited number of sites to which a calcium or phosphorus molecule can attach itself. Phosphorus competes with calcium for transport sites into the body; the more phosphorus you take in (particularly at the same meal in which calcium is being consumed), the less calcium you absorb. The less calcium you absorb, the more negative calcium balance, the slower bone growth, the faster your bone loss, and the greater your risk for osteoporosis.

The high-protein content of most American diets will also induce negative calcium balance. Exactly how this occurs is not entirely clear, but studies have shown that subjects fed a very high-protein diet will excrete more calcium in their urine than subjects fed a lower-protein diet. The most concentrated form of protein and phosphorus in our diet is meat. Thus, heavy meat eaters will be at increased risk for osteoporosis. Several studies have shown that vegetarians, particularly ovo-lactovegetarians, have more dense bones than meat eaters. In one study, bone density was greater in vegetarian women at age seventy than in fifty-year-old women who had consumed meat for most of their lives.

Finally, the large amount of salt ingested by most Americans has a negative effect on calcium balance. The excess sodium must be excreted by the kidneys. In this process extra calcium is also excreted. Thus, though the mechanism is indirect, the more sodium you consume, the more calcium you will lose and the higher your risk for osteoporosis.

Determining Your Risk Score

A score of 10 or above places either a woman or a man at high enough risk to alter the diet and increase the level of exercise. Since it is much easier for a woman to reach this score, many more women will find themselves at this risk level than men. However, for those men who score 10 or above, the dietary advice in the next section is just as important as for women.

Your Sex
As mentioned above, if you are a woman you are automatically at higher risk than if you are a man. All women therefore begin with a score of 5; all men with a score of 0.

Your Race
Racial tendencies toward osteoporosis pertain only to women, not to men. If you are a man, score 0 no matter what your race or ethnic background. If you are a black woman, score 0. If you are of Hispanic, Mediterranean, Eastern European, or Oriental background, score 1. If you are of northern European origin, or of extremely fair complexion, score 2.

Family History
If your mother or sister or several very close relatives have or have had osteoporosis, score 3. If a few aunts or cousins have or have had osteoporosis, score 2; if a scattering of distant relatives, 1; and if nobody in your family, 0.

Early Menopause
If you had a surgically induced menopause before natural menopause, score 5. If natural menopause occurred before age forty-five, score 3; if between age forty-five and

fifty-five, score 0. Thus, if you underwent surgical menopause before reaching the age of natural menopause, you
are automatically at high risk for osteoporosis. Even if you
are treated with estrogen, you should still start a program
of diet and exercise designed to prevent the disease.

Body Build
If you have a large frame and broad bones, score 0; an average frame, 1; and if you are petite and slight of build,
score 2.

Body Weight
Anyone of either sex who is 20 percent or more below
ideal weight increases his or her chances of developing
osteoporosis. If you fall into this category, score 2; between 10 and 20 percent, score 1. If your body weight is
above this figure (even if you are obese), score 0.

Oral Contraceptives
If you have been taking oral contraceptives for a long time
it has given you some protection against developing osteoporosis. How much protection is unclear. If you are such
an individual, subtract one point from your final score.
However, if this one point is the deciding factor between
whether or not to introduce preventive measures, it would
still be prudent to undertake those measures.

Number of Previous Pregnancies
If you have never been pregnant, score 3; if you have had
one pregnancy, score 1; more than one, score 0.

Breast-feeding
While breast-feeding one or more infants probably offers
you some protection, we do not know enough about it to
assign a risk score. However, there is certainly no reason
to be concerned that breast-feeding increases your risk. If

your calcium intake was adequate, you can expect an added bonus in lowering your score.

Exercise

If you have been bedridden or confined to a wheelchair for a long time (months or years), score 5; this is a very significant risk factor. Lesser periods of nonweight-bearing time should be scored proportionally. If you live a sedentary existence, score 2; take moderate but occasional exercise, score 1; engage in regular exercise, score 0.

Smoking

If you are a heavy cigarette smoker, score 1.

Alcohol

If you are an alcoholic, you need help for many reasons, only one of which is a higher risk for osteoporosis. Whether a man or a woman, if you fall into this category, score 5. If you are a woman, this score will automatically place you in the high-risk category. If you are a man, this score will send you well on your way. Heavy drinkers, even if they are not alcoholics, should score 3.

Medications

If you have taken cortisonelike drugs for a long time, score 5. This is a very significant risk factor and applies to both men and women. For shorter periods on these drugs, adjust your score appropriately, but remember those short periods can add up.

Anticonvulsant drugs will increase your risk but not as much as cortisone and its derivatives. Score 3 if you have been taking anticonvulsants for a long time.

Antacids also increase your risk. If you are a regular user of types that contain aluminum, score 2 (and change your brand if you cannot stop using them).

Illness

Whether a man or a woman, if you suffer from hyperparathyroidism, hyperthyroidism, or overactive adrenals (Cushing's syndrome), score 3. If you have diabetes, rheumatoid arthritis, or certain forms of kidney disease (ask your doctor which kinds), score 2.

Diet

If you are a vegetarian, particularly an ovo-lactovegetarian, score 0. If you eat the "typical" American diet, score 2. Heavy meat eaters should score 3. If you cannot or will not consume foods high in calcium (that is, if you have a lactose intolerance), score 3. If you are a constant dieter, taking in 1,200 calories or less, for long periods in your life, score 2.

You are now ready to calculate your risk score for osteoporosis. Table 22 lists various risk factors and their maximum scores. Fill in the column for your personal scores. If the total adds up to 10 or more, you are at high enough risk to institute preventive measures.

Examining the table you will see that if you are a woman, your chances for reaching a high-risk score of 10 or more are much greater than if you are a man. This is not surprising since osteoporosis is much more common in women than in men. For a woman, surgical menopause or severe alcoholism or chronic ingestion of cortisonelike drugs is enough to place her in the high-risk category. Men, however, can also be at high risk. For example, the heavy-drinking, very thin, slightly built man who smokes has a score of 10 and is at high risk. Similarly, a man with a strong family history of the disease, whose diet is poor, and who takes certain medications can also be at high risk.

The point scores allotted to the various categories have been assigned in such a way as to err on the side of overstatement of risk. This is because we cannot estimate risk precisely. Since preventive measures outlined in the next

TABLE 22

Risk Factor	Maximum Score	Your Score
Sex*	5	
Race or ethnic group*	2	
Family history	3	
Early menopause*	5	
Body build	2	
Body weight	2	
Previous pregnancies*	3	
Exercise	5	
Smoking	1	
Alcohol consumption	5	
Medications	5	
Illness	3	
Diet	3	
Total (women)	44	
(men)	29	

*Pertains to women only

section are without danger and have positive health benefits other than merely lowering your risk for osteoporosis, it would be prudent to institute them more often than not.

Lowering Your Risk

If your score is 10 or above, your risk for osteoporosis is great enough to undertake whatever preventive measures you can. At the same time, you may wish to undergo certain tests to determine actual bone density. These tests are available in many hospitals and involve newer forms of tissue-imaging that subject you to little or no radiation. They are helpful in determining if you have already undergone significant bone loss and for measuring the degree of probable success of any preventive measures you institute. They are not designed to influence your decision to begin preventive measures. Even though the tests may reveal normal bone mass, if your score is 10 or above, you should still begin a preventive program *before* significant bone loss has occurred. Subsequent tests will be able to tell you if your program is succeeding.

Examine your score carefully. Some of the risk factors are under your control and can be eliminated. Once these risk factors have been eliminated, to reduce your risk further, you will have to pay special attention to your diet and to the type and amount of physical activity you engage in.

A Diet to Lower Your Risk

The principles of a diet designed to lower your risk for osteoporosis include:

Adequate calories to attain and/or maintain ideal weight

A calcium intake of 1 gram (1,000 milligrams, or mg) per day; 1,500 mg during periods of high calcium need, such as adolescence, pregnancy, and lactation

A relatively low phosphorus intake

A relatively low protein intake

Avoidance of excess dietary sodium

Adequate but not excessive amounts of vitamin D

Calories

Calories are important for two reasons. If you are too thin your risk is increased. Additionally, you are unlikely to fulfill your calcium requirement if you are consuming too few calories.

Women who for cosmetic reasons are constantly taking in under 1,500 calories per day to maintain a weight that is 10 or 20 percent below their ideal weight are endangering their bones. We often hear about the problems of being overweight and assume that the thinner we are the better. Clearly, this is not true if you are at high risk for osteoporosis. Being too thin may be as much of a health risk as being too fat.

If you are truly obese, and at the same time are at increased risk for osteoporosis, you will want to follow the regimen outlined in Chapter 4 carefully. Avoid crash dieting or the use of fad diets. They are often very low in calcium. Emphasize foods of high nutrient density with specific attention to calcium. Choose foods of low-calorie and high-calcium content. For example, skim milk is much better than whole milk; low-fat yogurt is better than sour cream; cottage cheese is preferable to cream cheese. Finally, set realistic goals you can reach and maintain without constantly restricting calories to unrealistically low levels. If you are overweight but out of the danger zone, you will have reduced your risk for the complications of obesity. At the same time you will reap at least one benefit of being slightly overweight: your risk of developing osteoporosis will be lessened.

Dietary Calcium

The recommended dietary allowance for calcium (set by the Food and Nutrition Board of the National Academy of Sciences) for an adult woman is 800 mg per day and 1,200 mg per day during periods of increased calcium demand. I have recommended that the amounts be slightly higher (see the principles outlined above) because women who are at risk for osteoporosis often begin with a deficit. The levels I have set, however, are attainable by eating a proper diet and calcium supplements are necessary only if you cannot or will not consume adequate amounts of high-calcium foods.

Table 23 lists foods high in calcium and their actual calcium content per average serving.

You can see that most of the high-calcium foods fall into

TABLE 23   Calcium Content of Foods
*(each portion provides approximately
300 mg of calcium)*

Food	Amount
Almonds	1 cup
Amaranth	4 oz.
Broccoli	2¼ cups
Cheese:	
cottage	12 oz.
sandwich-style	1½ to 2 oz.
Custard	1 cup
Fish (canned):*	
mackerel	3½ oz.
salmon	5½ oz.
sardines	3½ oz.
Ice cream (regular)	1⅔ cup
Kelp	1½ oz.
Milk:	
whole, low-fat, or	
buttermilk	8 oz.
Tofu (soybean curd)	8 oz.
Tortillas (6 in. diam.)	5
Yeast (brewers')	14 tbsp.
Yogurt	¾–⅘ cup

*This calcium level includes the softened bones. If the bones
are discarded the calcium content is greatly reduced.

the category of dairy products (Americans normally get
about 80 percent of their calcium from dairy products).
However, by making careful food choices you can get the
required amount of calcium with a much lower percentage coming from milk and milk products. For example, any
daily menu that includes single portions of any two of the
following: almonds, broccoli, canned fish (with bones),
kelp, tofu, tortillas, kale, turnip or collard greens, maca-
roni and cheese, pizza, beef tacos, or cheese or meat
enchiladas will supply more than half your calcium

requirement. Although the rest of your diet will supply some calcium, still you will generally need some dairy foods to reach your requirement. If you cannot eat any dairy products you should take a calcium supplement. A more complete discussion of the use of calcium supplements will follow.

Dietary Phosphorus

A diet high in phosphorus will inhibit adequate calcium absorption and thereby effectively reduce the amount of calcium getting into your body. For optimal calcium absorption you should strive for a dietary pattern that gives you twice as much calcium as phosphorus. This will probably entail some changes in your diet, since the average American consumes more phosphorus than calcium. The major dietary sources of phosphorus are meat, particularly red meat, and for some people, carbonated soft drinks. These foods contain very little calcium. Thus, the calcium-phosphorus ratio, which should be 2:1, is very low. Foods such as beef liver, bologna, fried chicken, corn on the cob, frankfurters, ground beef, ham, lamb chops, and pork chops have a calcium-phosphorus ratio from 1:15 to 1:45. Some of the phosphorylated soft drinks contain almost no calcium. By contrast, many green leafy vegetables, such as spinach and lettuce, have more calcium than phosphorus and hence have a favorable calcium-phosphorus ratio. Dairy products, which are high in calcium, also contain significant amounts of phosphorus, and their calcium-phosphorus ratio, although favorable, is not as good as that of some of the plant foods.

From a practical standpoint, what this means is that a diet to lower your risk for osteoporosis should not only be high in calcium but also be low in phosphorus. Anytime you can include foods that satisfy both these criteria, you are ahead of the game.

Table 24 is a list of high-phosphorus foods and the average phosphorus content per serving.

TABLE 24   Phosphorus Content of Foods

Food	Weight	MgP
Beef liver	3 oz.	405
Calf's liver	3 oz.	456
Lean beef	3 oz.	207
Chicken, light	3½ oz.	280
Chicken, dark	3 oz.	188
Pork, lean	3 oz.	185
Egg, large	1 (57 grams)	103
Milk, whole	8 oz.	227
Milk, 2% fat	8 oz.	276
Milk, skim	8 oz.	233
Cottage cheese, creamed	1 cup (210 grams)	319
Cheddar cheese	1 oz. (28 grams)	136
Bread, whole wheat	1 slice (28 grams)	71
Bread, white	1 slice (28 grams)	28
Peanuts	1 oz.	114
Kidney beans	1 cup (185 grams)	259
Almonds	1 oz.	143

In addition to the overall content of calcium and phosphorus in your diet, the time you eat these two nutrients in relation to each other is very important. Because calcium and phosphorus compete for the binding sites on the transport protein ("seats on the train"), the more you separate the intake of these two minerals, the better. The calcium from the sour cream in your baked-potato-and-steak meal is not absorbed as well as the calcium from your late evening ice-cream snack. The meals that emphasize calcium-rich foods are better absorbed if phosphorus-rich foods are avoided. A good idea would be to emphasize calcium-rich snack foods, which are often eaten by themselves.

Protein
The very high-protein diets consumed by most Americans will result in more calcium being excreted in their urine

than occurs in people who consume less protein. Like phosphorus, the main source of dietary protein is meat. The more meat you eat, the more calcium you lose, and the greater your risk for osteoporosis. This does not mean that you have to eliminate meat. It does mean, however, that you should use moderation. Every meal does not have to contain meat. Try to limit your meat intake to one meal a day, and cut down on the size of your portions. Emphasize calcium at other meals and during snacks. Remember, if you are consuming dairy products to supply calcium, you will automatically be getting significant amounts of protein and need not worry about protein deficiency.

Vegetarians, particularly ovo-lactovegetarians, have a lower incidence of osteoporosis than meat eaters. This is probably because of the lower protein and phosphorus content of their diets. A well-balanced vegetarian diet that allows milk and milk products is probably best for preventing osteoporosis. The closer you approximate such a diet, the better. However, a pure vegetarian, or vegan, diet (no meat, milk products, or eggs) can be a problem unless nondairy sources of calcium are provided. A vegetarian diet has the advantages of affording good calcium absorption and low calcium excretion; therefore, the actual calcium requirement is probably considerably less than on the typical American diet. However, even with these factors in your favor, if your risk for osteoporosis is high you must pay special attention to your calcium intake. Diets which claim to be variations of vegetarianism but are much more restrictive—for example, macrobiotic diets—will *increase* your risk for osteoporosis. They will be too low in calcium to supply your body's needs, and should be discouraged for several reasons, not the least of which is their tendency to increase your risk for osteoporosis.

Sodium
A very high-salt intake will force your kidneys to excrete more sodium. In the process, calcium will be excreted.

You do not have to go on a low-sodium diet to protect your bones from osteoporosis, but if you are a saltaholic, you should cut back. The mild sodium restriction described in Chapter 3 is not very limiting and will not place an excessive load on your kidneys. An occasional transgression can be tolerated without endangering your bones. Remember the nondietary sources of sodium, such as over-the-counter medications, and avoid them when possible.

Vitamin D
Most American diets, particularly those adequate in calcium, will be adequate in vitamin D. Thus, a diet for preventing osteoporosis should almost always have enough of this important vitamin. However, most of our dietary vitamin D comes from dairy products made from milk that has been fortified. If you cannot take more than small amounts of these foods, you may have to eat other foods that have been fortified or take a supplement. Remember, vitamin D in excess amounts can be very dangerous, and since it is stored in the body, its effects can be cumulative. If you must take a supplement, take no more than the RDA (400 IU).

Calcium Supplements

There are two advantages to taking a calcium supplement if you are at risk for osteoporosis:

You can guarantee an adequate amount of calcium for your body's needs.

You can consume the calcium in a form and at a time that will promote maximum absorption.

Since there is no known toxicity for moderate doses of calcium supplements even when they are taken for a long time, I have no objection to using a supplement *as·an added protection* for anyone at risk for osteoporosis. If your diet makes it difficult for you to get enough calcium, if you are an avid meat eater, if you cannot do without phosphorylated soft drinks, then you must take a calcium supplement. If your risk score is 15 or above, I would also recommend a calcium supplement. If you cannot give up heavy drinking, you should take a calcium supplement, and if you are constantly cutting calories, a supplement also will ensure that you get enough. One gram per day is more than adequate for your needs.

As you can see, I am advocating that most people at risk for osteoporosis take a daily calcium supplement. If your score is between 10 and 15 and you are able to eat foods that are high in calcium and moderately low in phosphorus and protein, a calcium supplement is optional. If your score is 15 or above, or if you are a heavy user of alcohol, then a calcium supplement should be taken. The best time to take this supplement is between meals to minimize the dietary factors that interfere with calcium absorption.

The use of a calcium supplement is to ensure that you get enough total calcium; it should not be used as a replacement for a high calcium diet. At present the evidence indicates that a *diet* high in calcium and low in phosphorus and protein offers some protection from osteoporosis. There is no evidence that calcium supplements can *replace* such a diet. In addition, dietary patterns become a habit. If you can establish a pattern that emphasizes high calcium, low protein, and low phosphorus, you will be able to maintain such a diet for the rest of your life. This is extremely important if you wish to minimize your risk for osteoporosis.

Any of the calcium supplements that are available can be used with the exception of calcium phosphate. Calcium carbonate is usually the cheapest and contains the most calcium per tablet. Calcium lactate should be avoided by people who are lactose intolerant. Calcium gluconate contains only small amounts of calcium per tablet and hence must be taken several times during the day. Calcium chloride irritates the stomach in some people. Bone meal and dolomite are high in calcium but contain significant amounts of phosphorus and may be contaminated by toxic substances; hence they are not as good as the purer tablets.

Whichever form of supplement you choose, establish a routine and take it at the same time every day.

Exercise

Exercise is important for maintaining healthy bones and is particularly important if you are at high risk for osteoporosis. The best kind of exercise will combine movement and stress on the long bones. Walking, bicycling, hiking, jogging, rowing, and gymnastics are all excellent. But even more important than undertaking a specific exercise program is maintaining an active life-style. Walk when you can, climb that flight of stairs, stand rather than sit. Let your bones do their job of bearing the weight of your body. If you do all these things, you will lower your risk for osteoporosis.

Too much exercise, particularly for young women, may actually increase the risk for osteoporosis. Although the number of women athletes studied is still small, results of tests suggest that exercising to the point where menstruation ceases may increase the risk of bone loss.

It is difficult to say how much exercise is enough. However, a regime used for promoting cardiovascular fitness is certainly adequate. Since most people will benefit from such a regime, you may well derive a double benefit.

Deciding if Your Risk Is Improving

It is important for anyone who is at risk for osteoporosis to have bone mass assessed at regular intervals. For most, the program outlined above will show tangible results in that bone mass will stay the same or regress very slowly. The tests will serve to reenforce your diet and exercise program and give you an incentive to keep up the good work. For some, however, even if the nutrition and exercise program is diligently adhered to, bone loss will progress. At this point you have to make a difficult decision in consultation with your physician whether to institute estrogen therapy.

The Use of Estrogens

There is no question that estrogen therapy can prevent the bone loss that accompanies removal of the ovaries or natural menopause. It is the most effective treatment currently available, and it is the only effective treatment that can be undertaken if the dietary and exercise regime outlined above is not slowing the rate of bone loss adequately. To be effective, estrogen therapy must continue for a long time (ten to fifteen years). Since this treatment will increase your risk for cancer of the uterus, and perhaps of the breast, it is not a decision to be taken lightly. However, progressive osteoporosis is a very serious problem, which can lead to death and disabilities if severe fractures occur. Thus, the decision you are faced with is balancing the risk of using estrogen against the risk of not using it.

Let us examine these two risks carefully. The incidence of cancer of the uterus among the general population is about one per thousand. The use of estrogen after menopause increases that risk four to eight times. Therefore, at most, if you undertake estrogen treatment, your risk for developing cancer of the uterus is eight per thousand. Of 1,000 women taking estrogen, 992 will *not* get uterine cancer. The evidence for breast cancer is not conclusive. Some studies suggest a slight increase with estrogen treatment, some suggest no change in incidence, and some even suggest a decrease in incidence. Present evidence suggests that women with a family history of breast cancer, or with other known risk factors for the disease (see Chapter 6), will have their risk increased by long-term estrogen treatment. Just how much of an increase is not clear. Using the best data available, it appears that if we use estrogen therapy only in women who show no known risk factors for either breast or uterine cancer, this will increase their risk of uterine cancer from one per thousand to, at most, eight per thousand, and will not increase their risk of breast cancer significantly.

Balanced against these numbers is the risk of developing severe osteoporosis and its potentially debilitating fractures. In some cases the decision is clear. Almost all physicians will treat surgically induced premenopausal removal of the ovaries with estrogen. Rapid bone loss in the face of dietary treatment is also an indication for treatment. But how rapid is rapid? Only a physician trained in this area is qualified to make such a decision. In the last analysis you will have to rely on your physician's judgment and that is how it should be. However, now you know what questions to ask, and you can take some consolation in knowing that even if a decision is made to start estrogen therapy, your risk of cancer in actual numbers is really very small. In addition, your physician may elect to use progesterone together with estrogen, which may reduce your cancer risk even further. Perhaps nowhere in the entire area of disease prevention are the training, experience, and judgment of your physician more important than in helping you decide whether to use estrogen treatment to prevent osteoporosis.

Here is a summary of the most important steps you can take to protect yourself from osteoporosis:

Calculate your risk score. If it is below 10, stay alert but you need not take specific measures. If your score is 10 or above, take the following steps:

Eliminate those factors under your control (alcohol, smoking, certain drugs).

Have your bone mass measured periodically.

Consume a diet of adequate calories to reach or maintain ideal weight; one that is high in calcium, low in phosphorus and protein, and not excessive in salt.

Undertake regular activities and an exercise program that will place modest stress on your bones.

Take a calcium supplement (optional for scores 10 to 15; mandatory for scores of 15 and above).

If your bone mass continues to decrease rapidly even when the above measures have been instituted:

Discuss with your physician the pros and cons of estrogen treatment and decide whether such treatment would be best for you.

Chapter 9

Double Jeopardy

Clearly, being at risk for one of the diseases we have discussed does not preclude the possibility that you are at risk for another. In fact, with certain of them, being at risk for one increases your chances of being at risk for another. People at risk for obesity are more likely to be at risk for high blood pressure, high blood levels of fat, and diabetes. In some cases all these diseases seem to run in the same kinds of families. Certain environments and dietary factors are common among all of them. It is no surprise, therefore, that many people are at risk for more than one disease. If your risk scores show you at high risk for more than one disease, how should you handle this? Can a diet to prevent obesity be modified also to protect you against hypertension or diabetes or atherosclerosis? The answer is yes. No matter what combination of risks you have, you can undertake a diet that is not overly restrictive and can offer you maximum protection against all the diseases for which your risk is high. In this chapter, I will point out those combinations that are likely to go together and the dietary principles that should be considered when you make your actual food choices.

Classification of Diseases: Overabundance and Deficiency

Essentially there are two kinds of dietary manipulations that can reduce your risk for the diseases discussed earlier. There are those diseases in which *too much* of a particular nutrient or combination of nutrients increases your risk and there are those in which *too little* does. Atherosclerosis, hypertension, obesity, diabetes, and cancer are more likely to occur if you consume too much; osteoporosis and anemia if you consume too little. Thus, to lower your risk for any disease in the first group, you must *restrict* your intake of certain nutrients. To lower your risk for osteoporosis and anemia, you must *increase* your intake for certain nutrients. Fortunately, no nutrient that must be reduced to protect you against one illness must be increased to protect you against another. Thus, a satisfactory diet can be easily constructed no matter for how many of these illnesses your risk score is high.

If we examine the nutrients that must be altered to reduce your risk for all these diseases, the number is small: seven—calories, fat, salt (sodium), calcium, iron, zinc, and folic acid. In fact, a diet low in calories, fat, and salt, and high in calcium, iron, zinc, and folic acid would protect you against all of the diseases. Such a diet is not only quite reasonable, but some nutrition experts advise that *all* Americans consume it to lower their risk of all the diseases discussed.

However, I have been saying that not *everyone* has to change his or her diet this way. That the major benefits to be derived from any of these dietary changes are specific to individuals at high risk for a certain disease. There is no reason to institute a particular dietary change that might be of benefit statistically if everyone made it, if it would be of little benefit to you. However, it should be pointed out that a regimen such as the type advocated above is not only healthy for everyone, but can usually be achieved without major inconvenience. Certainly, therefore, anyone at risk for more than one disease can change his or her diet and simultaneously lower all the risks. Instituting *all* these changes is rarely necessary, since those who are at risk for one disease influenced by *excessive* intake will probably be at risk for another influenced by excessive intake. By contrast, those who are prone to one disease influenced by deficient nutrient intake will be prone to the other disease similarly influenced. This is true for several reasons. First, the genetic factors that increase risk for atherosclerosis, obesity, hypertension, and diabetes seem to be linked in some way. Second, the diseases of nutrient deficiencies, osteoporosis and anemia, occur almost exclusively in women. Finally, the life-styles of most people generally place them in one group (in which excesses must be avoided) or the other (in which deficiencies must be corrected), but rarely in both. Let us therefore examine these groups from the standpoint of someone at risk for more than one disease.

Too Much

The diseases in this group are atherosclerosis, hypertension, obesity, diabetes, and certain cancers. The nutrients are calories, fat, and salt consumed in excessive amounts. Salt (sodium) is specific for hypertension. Thus, if the combination of diseases for which your score was high included hypertension, you must limit your salt intake as outlined in the chapter on hypertension. Calories and fat are inextricably linked. Fat is the most calorie-dense nutrient and hence the major source of excessive calories. Therefore, reducing calories almost always means reducing fat, and reducing fat invariably means reducing calories. For practical purposes, for all these diseases you must reduce the amount of fat in your diet whether you are aiming primarily at fat reduction, as in atherosclerosis and cancer; or calorie reduction, as in hypertension or obesity; or both, as in diabetes. Once you have done this, you can focus on the calories independent of the fat you take 'n. Hence, if calories are of primary concern, you may wish to cut them down further by reducing your intake of alcohol and refined sugar, and in some cases by reducing your overall intake of food. The steps to be taken if you are at risk for more than one of the diseases in this group are as follows:

• Reduce the amount of total fat (for any combination of diseases).

• Reduce calories further (for obesity, hypertension, diabetes).

• Reduce sodium (for hypertension).

You can see that the most restrictive diet is the one for hypertension, which attempts to control sodium and calories. By reducing fat as discussed in the chapter on atherosclerosis, you will help bring calories into balance. Thus, by only slightly modifying the diet for those at risk for hypertension, you will be protecting yourself from any combination of diseases. If your risk for hypertension is not increased, then no matter what the combined diseases are, you do not have to pay specific attention to salt reduction.

Too Little
In this group are two diseases, osteoporosis and anemia. Both primarily concern women, and a considerable number of American women may be at risk for both. A woman at high risk for osteoporosis and anemia must pay particular attention to consuming foods with a high calcium, iron, zinc, and folic acid content. At the same time, she should limit her phosphorus intake particularly at the same meal that supplies a considerable portion of her calcium intake. This type of diet, of all those discussed, probably de-

mands the greatest knowledge of the specific nutrients in foods. As we have noted, dietary calcium comes primarily from dairy foods. Fat-free or low-fat dairy foods are more nutrient-dense and hence allow you to take in other caloric sources of necessary iron, zinc, and folic acid. Folic acid and zinc requirements have risen only moderately and the inclusion of *lean* meat, liver, seafood, and certain green leafy vegetables in generous amounts should meet this increased requirement. As for iron, a risk score above 10 should be treated initially with iron supplements if you are at double risk. This must be done because to satisfy your calcium requirement, you will be consuming foods that are low in iron (milk, cheese, yogurt, etc.). Thus, you must get your iron from only a part of your diet. If your iron requirement is very high, then it can be achieved effectively only by consuming fortified foods (which also supply calories) or by taking an iron supplement. Conversely, meat is not a particularly good source of calcium and is high in phosphorus. Therefore, a diet that emphasizes meat reduces the availability and the absorption of calcium. Unless you eat dairy products and carefully selected plant foods (see Table 23, page 218), you will have difficulty getting your calcium requirement. In that case, you should take a calcium supplement. The following guidelines should be followed if you are at risk for both osteoporosis and anemia:

- Choose foods rich in calcium, iron, zinc, and folic acid, and low in calories.
- Use low-fat dairy products.
- Favor nondairy sources of calcium that also contain significant quantities of iron, zinc, or folic acid.
- Use fortified breakfast cereals that contain iron primarily, and folic acid and zinc when possible.
- Take a calcium supplement if you cannot achieve your calcium requirement (1,000 to 1,200 mg per day) with

the above diet. This will depend on the number of calories you are consuming.

- Take an iron supplement if your risk score for anemia is 10 or more.
- If you are deliberately limiting calories (dieting), take a calcium supplement (500 to 1,000 mg per day) and an iron supplement (30 mg per day).

Essentially what you are trying to do is combine a diet that lowers your risk for osteoporosis with one designed to lower your risk for anemia. This can be achieved effectively only if you take in enough food (calories) of the proper nutrient density, and if your iron reserves are not too badly depleted. Otherwise, you should take a calcium supplement, an iron supplement, or both.

Too Much and Too Little

Occasionally someone, usually a woman, can be at simultaneous risk for one disease from the nutrient-excess group and one from the nutrient-deficient group. For example, a woman may be at risk for hypertension and anemia. If so, she must keep her weight down by controlling calories, reduce her salt intake, and increase her intake of iron, zinc, and folic acid. To do this, she must pay attention to the foods in her diet. First, the calories: how many can she take in without exceeding her ideal weight? If the number is below 1,800, she will have a problem getting her iron requirement; below 1,200, she will need an iron supplement no matter how careful she is about her diet. Second, she must pay special attention to the sources of zinc, folic acid, and iron (see Tables 18 to 20, Chapter 7). Finally, she must avoid foods that are either naturally high in sodium or to which sodium has been added.

If cholesterol and saturated fat have to be reduced, then your options for iron become fewer since this means reducing your intake of red meats and organ meats, the richest sources of this mineral. Because it may be difficult to get all the nutrients you need, if you are in double jeopardy for a deficiency disease and a disease of excess you should consider taking supplements. This will allow you to concentrate on lowering your risk for atherosclerosis, hypertension, obesity, diabetes, or certain cancers while protecting yourself against osteoporosis or anemia. Taking supplements, however, does not mean that you need not emphasize dietary sources of iron, zinc, folic acid, and calcium. The best way to get these nutrients is from your food; the supplements are simply insurance. For those of you at risk for diseases of both excess and deficiency, the following principles should be observed·

- Decide how many calories you need.
- Reduce calories, fat, and salt as dictated by your risk in the excess category.
- Increase foods as needed if you are in the deficient category.
- Take a supplement—iron if you are at risk for anemia, calcium if you are at risk for osteoporosis, iron and calcium if you are at risk for both diseases.

Nutritional Supplements
There is only one reason to take nutritional supplements—you are unable to get your nutritional requirement from your diet alone. As we have seen, this is rarely a problem for adult men. By contrast, adult women may need supplements under certain conditions. We have already seen some of these conditions:

- High-risk score for nutritional anemia (iron)
- Risk for osteoporosis; inability to consume large amounts of dairy foods (calcium)
- Pregnancy (iron and folic acid)
- Adolescent pregnancy (iron, folic acid, zinc [calcium])

- Any risk score for anemia in a pure vegetarian (iron, zinc, and vitamin B_{12})
- Risk for osteoporosis and one of the diseases of excess (calcium)
- Risk for anemia and one of the diseases of excess (iron)
- Risk for osteoporosis, anemia, and one of the diseases of excess (iron and calcium)
- Any woman consuming less than 1,200 calories (iron)
- Risk for anemia; heavy alcohol consumption (iron, zinc, and folic acid)

Nutrient supplements can be gotten by consuming fortified foods or by taking a pill containing vitamins and minerals. The former supplies the nutrients with some calories (usually from carbohydrates); the latter has no calories. Whichever type you choose remember you are taking a supplement for a reason: your diet is low in that particular nutrient. Therefore, decide which supplement you need (use the chart above), and then pick a fortified food or pill containing it. For example, if you need iron and decide to use a fortified breakfast cereal, which brand should you choose? Brand X contains 100 percent of the daily requirement for all the vitamins and 25 percent of the daily requirement of iron. Brand Y contains only 25 to 50 percent of the vitamins, but 35 percent of the daily iron requirement. Brand Y should be your choice even though it is not as high in vitamins. On the other hand, if you need both iron and folic acid, you might elect Brand X, which has 100 percent of the folic acid. Simply look for the highest amount of the nutrient or nutrients you need. Don't be fooled by ads saying that one cereal provides better nutrition than another cereal because it contains more of certain nutrients if you do not need those nutrients.

The same principle holds if you decide to use pills. Pick one that has the right amount of the nutrient you need.

The rest of the vitamins and minerals it contains are unnecessary. For example, if you need 30 mg of iron per day,
take a pill that contains 30 mg of iron. The amount of B-
complex vitamins or vitamins C or A or D the pill contains is unimportant; in fact, taking too much of some of
these unnecessary nutrients can be dangerous. If you need
only iron, then take only iron. If you need iron and folic
acid or zinc, you may wish to take a multivitamin mineral
preparation. Ideally you should take only one pill that
contains all three nutrients in the right amounts. Unfortunately such a pill might not exist. Therefore, select a pill
with as much of these three nutrients as you need and with
as few of the others as possible. In particular, avoid pills
that are very high in vitamins A and D, since these nutrients may be toxic if taken in excessive amounts.

If you need calcium, you cannot use fortified foods since
none contain sufficient amounts. You will need to take your
calcium in pill form. In general, you should use one pill
for calcium and another for iron, zinc, and folic acid if you
need all four nutrients, since pills containing both calcium and the others are not usually available. In the chapter on osteoporosis, I discussed the best type of calcium
pills to take.

Being in "double jeopardy" can be handled with a minimum of inconvenience. For most, it will mean a somewhat more restricted diet. For a few, it will mean taking
supplements too. Look at the diets that lower your risk
for the particular diseases in question. What you will want
to do is combine them. Make a list of the foods you have
to *avoid* in each disease. For example, if you are at risk
for atherosclerosis and hypertension, you will want to avoid
fatty meats, organ meats, eggs, nonskimmed dairy products (atherosclerosis), and luncheon meats, hot dogs, etc.
(atherosclerosis and hypertension), and pickled, smoked,
and highly processed foods (hypertension). In addition, you
will not be adding much salt during cooking or using the
salt shaker at the table. Somewhat restrictive? Of course.

You are at risk for two serious diseases! But there is an endless variety of foods you can eat: fish, fowl, lean meats, skim dairy products, fruits, vegetables, starches, grains, even wine or other alcoholic beverages in moderation. If you are at risk for obesity, this diet will be low in calories; if you are at risk for breast cancer or uterine cancer, the lowered fat and calories will reduce your risk; if your diabetes score is high, the diet will also reduce your risk.

If you are at risk for one or more of these diseases and are also at risk for osteoporosis or anemia, you must choose wisely from among the foods that are permitted. In addition, take a calcium supplement for osteoporosis or an iron supplement if your risk for anemia is high. Finally, if you are at high risk for atherosclerosis, hypertension, obesity, or osteoporosis, you may want to increase your exercise level, particularly if you tend to be inactive. All the changes I am recommending are consistent with today's more active life-style and can be accomplished without great difficulty. You can continue to prepare gourmet meals at home and to dine in fine restaurants. In fact, some of the finest restaurants now offer choices consistent with the principles I have outlined above. So even for those at risk for two or more diseases, there is plenty of room to enjoy good food. Just be aware and choose wisely. You have everything to gain and very little to lose.

Chapter 10

When Risk Cannot Be Determined

It would be nice if we could develop a precise risk score for each nutritionally related disease so that a person could determine his or her own risk and decide whether or not a dietary change will be of personal benefit. Unfortunately, this cannot be done with precision in most diseases with which we are concerned. In some, like the ones we have discussed, we can at least define certain genetic and life-style characteristics that will predispose an individual to a particular disease. If these predisposing factors are numerous enough to raise your risk score above a certain number, you must consider modifying your diet. If your risk score is low, dietary modification is probably not necessary. In other diseases, however, we know there is an association with diet, but we do not have enough information to develop a risk profile. For example, diverticulosis is associated with a diet low in fiber, but we are not able to separate people at high risk from those at low risk. Any recommendations we make for diseases that fit into this category will be for the general public. They will depend on two factors, the prevalence of the disease and your own dietary practices.

Let me illustrate what I mean. Suppose there is a disease that affects 20 percent of the population; you have one chance in five of developing it. If your diet puts you in the category of being more prone to this disease, you may want to change it. By contrast, let us suppose the disease in question has an incidence of 1 percent or less. Your chances for getting it are less than one in a hundred. You may elect not to change your diet. Not only will the incidence of the disease influence your choice, but its severity is also important. You may elect to take a one-in-a-hundred chance for one disease, but not for another. In this chapter I will discuss a number of serious diseases that are associated with diet and for which a risk profile cannot be defined. I will try to give you a description of the disease and to outline its prevalence. I will describe the kind of dietary practices associated with the disease. If you have these eating habits, you may want to change them. The decision is up to you! For those of you who elect to make a change, I will try to describe the best way to accomplish it.

Diseases of the Large Intestine

The gastrointestinal tract is divided into four discrete regions. The esophagus is a tube passing from the mouth through the thorax and diaphragm to the stomach. It is essentially a tunnel through which the food passes, helped along by muscular contractions that propel the food in the proper direction. The stomach is a bag that mixes the food and begins the process of digestion. The small intestine is a very long, relatively narrow coiled tube in which most digestion and absorption of food takes place. And the large intestine is a relatively short, wide tube in which water is reabsorbed and the undigested food is processed for excretion. Disease that occurs anywhere along this lengthy tract will often call for a change in diet, since the type and consistency of the food passing through may aggravate or ameliorate the condition. In addition, certain diseases within the gastrointestinal tract, particularly in the small intestine, may affect digestion or absorption of specific nutrients, and thereby necessitate a change in diet or the use of a dietary supplement. In this chapter we are not concerned with this type of disease because although diet is part of the treatment, sometimes the major part, it is not related to the cause of the disease. If you have such a condition you should be under a physician's care.

There are diseases of the gastrointestinal tract, particularly of the large intestine, which may be *caused* by improper diet over a long period of time. To understand how diet may cause these diseases, we must take a more careful look at what happens to the residue of our food as it traverses the large intestine. Very little absorption or digestion takes place after the food enters the large intestine. It is simply being prepared for excretion. The consistency of the food residue within the large intestine and the amount of pressure that must be generated to expel this material depends to a large extent on what the undigested residue reaching the large intestine consists of. When we eat we consume certain complex carbohydrates that we are unable to digest. These pass intact through the entire system and reach the large intestine in virtually the same condition as when eaten. This undigested complex carbohydrate is called fiber. It comes from cereal brans and from various fruits and vegetables. While there are many different types of fiber, they all have one property in common: they trap water. The more fiber in the diet, the more water in the material passing through the large intestines. The more water, the softer the material and, ultimately, the softer the stool. Thus, one way to prevent constipation (or, for that matter, to treat constipation) is to consume a high-fiber diet. Constipation can be a serious problem for many, particularly older people.

By creating a softer stool, a high-fiber diet will affect the large intestine in two ways. First, it will reduce the amount of pressure necessary to move the stool along for ultimate excretion. And second, a high-fiber diet moves the contents of the large intestine rapidly and generates less pressure while doing it.

The large intestine is a muscular tube lined inside with specialized cells. Normally there are stronger and weaker areas in the tube, and if very high pressure is constantly being generated within the tube, some of these areas will balloon and form small outpouchings called diverticuli. If many outpouchings form, we call the condition diverticulosis. Diverticulosis is much more common in older people. Twenty percent or more people over sixty-five may have diverticulosis. This is not surprising, since it is high pressure over a long time that causes the problem. Occasionally food or other debris within the large intestine gets trapped inside one or more of these diverticuli. This creates conditions that favor infection and the diverticuli become inflamed. When this happens, we term the condition diverticulitis. Diverticulitis is painful and serious, and demands immediate medical attention.

We don't know what makes one person more prone to developing diverticuli than another. Perhaps minute differences in the nature of the intestinal wall itself cause them. We do know, however, that increasing the amount of fiber in the diet reduces the risk of diverticulosis and its most serious consequence, diverticulitis.

Should you go on a higher-fiber diet? That depends on how much fiber you are consuming. Table 25 lists foods that are high in fiber. How often do you eat these foods?

In general, natural foods are higher in fiber than processed foods, and plant foods are higher in fiber than animal foods. Thus, the closer you are to being a vegetarian, the higher the fiber content of your diet.

Before you decide whether you need more fiber, you should consider another disease that may be related to a low-fiber diet. This disease is much less common than diverticulosis but much more serious: cancer of the colon. It is the second property of fiber in the diet that appears to protect against cancer of the colon or the large

TABLE 25   Fiber Content of Some Common Foods

Food	Amount (Measure)	Fiber (G)
Almonds	½ cup	1.8
Apple, unpeeled	1 medium	1.5
Asparagus pieces, cooked	½ cup	0.3
Bananas	1 medium	0.9
Beans, green, cooked	½ cup	0.6
Bran, wheat	2 tsp.	1.0–2.0
Bread, white or French	2 slices	0.1
Bread, whole wheat	2 slices	0.9
Broccoli, chopped, cooked	½ cup	1.2
Bulgur wheat, cooked	½ cup	0.5
Cabbage, cooked	½ cup	0.6
Cabbage, raw, shredded	½ cup	0.3
Carrots, cooked	½ cup	0.7
Carrots, raw	1 medium	0.5
Celery	1 stalk	0.3
Corn on cob, cooked	1 ear	1.0
Cornflakes	1 cup	0.2
Cucumber	½ medium	0.8
Lettuce, iceberg	⅛ head	0.3
Lettuce, romaine	2 leaves	0.4
Macaroni, cooked	½ cup	0.1
Mushrooms	10 small	0.8
Noodles, cooked	½ cup	0.1
Oatmeal, cooked	½ cup	0.2
Orange	1 medium	0.9
Orange juice	½ cup	0.1
Peanuts, roasted	½ cup	1.7
Peas, cooked	½ cup	− 0.5
Popcorn	3 oz.	2.0
Potatoes, baked in skin	1 medium	0.6
Potatoes, mashed	½ cup	0.4
Rice, brown, cooked	½ cup	0.3
Rice, white, cooked	½ cup	0.1
Soybeans, cooked	½ cup	1.0
Spinach, cooked	½ cup	0.5
Squash, summer, cooked	½ cup	0.6

Food	Amount (Measure)	Fiber (G)
Squash, winter, cooked	½ cup	1.4
Strawberries, raw	½ cup	1.0
Tomato	1 medium	0.8
Walnuts	½ cup	1.1

intestines. The more fiber in the diet, the faster the intestinal contents move, the less chance they have to come in contact with the intestinal wall. If there are substances within the stool that can induce cancer, the exposure time to such substances is reduced on a high-fiber diet. Whether such substances are actually present in the contents of the large intestine appears also in part to depend on the nature of your diet. The higher its fat content, the higher the risk for colon cancer. Thus, the best type of diet to reduce your risk for colon cancer is one high in fiber and low in fat. Our primary dietary sources of fat are meat and dairy products. These foods, as we have seen, are also low in fiber. By *increasing* the amount of fiber in your diet, you will almost automatically *decrease* the amount of fat.

We can summarize the arguments for a high-fiber diet as follows:

- It will keep the stool soft and help prevent constipation.

- It will keep the pressure inside the large intestine low and reduce the risk of diverticulosis.

- It will move the contents of the large intestine more rapidly, reducing contact time with the intestinal wall. And it will almost always reduce the amount of fat in the diet, thereby reducing the potential carcinogen content of the stool.

These effects, taken together, will reduce your risk for cancer of the colon.

How do you know if your diet contains enough fiber? The average American diet contains about 5 grams of fiber per day. Most authorities believe that the optimal amount of dietary fiber is about 15 grams of fiber. Look at Table 23. Add up the amount of fiber that you consume on an average day. Try to increase your consumption of high-fiber foods to approach 15 grams. You may find by doing this that the quantity of food you are consuming may increase to the extent that you can't eat it all. Good! Cut back on some of the high-fat foods in your diet.

If you plan to undertake this type of dietary change, do it gradually. If you suddenly begin to take in much more fiber than you are used to, you may feel bloated and suffer from gas pains. Your gastrointestinal tract needs time to adapt to the higher-fiber content in the foods it must process. Make the change over several weeks, progressively increasing your fiber intake by small amounts each day.

Disease of the Teeth

One of the great fears of getting old is the prospect of losing one's teeth. One out of every five of our older population has lost all teeth. There is increasing evidence that faulty nutrition plays some role in causing this problem. In early life, diet is related to dental caries; in later life, it is related to periodontal disease.

Dental Caries

There is no doubt that dental caries are related to diet. Specifically there is a strong association between the amount of refined sugar in our diet and the incidence of dental caries. To understand the nature of this relationship, we must examine in some detail how cavities occur.

The mouth is normally a breeding ground for millions of bacteria. The conditions within the mouth as well as the food eaten favor the growth of certain types of bacteria. Some of these organisms break down simple sugars, such as sucrose (ordinary refined sugar), to a number of products, including organic acids, and also use these sugars to construct a hard substance, called dental plaque, which adheres to the teeth. Thus, a diet high in simple sugar favors the growth of bacteria that require simple sugars to live. These bacteria, in turn, metabolize the simple sugar in a way that releases products which cause dental caries.

The process works like this. The bacteria secrete substances that form plaque. The plaque adheres to the teeth, and the bacteria hiding beneath it are sheltered from your toothbrush. These bacteria continue to break down the simple sugar and in the process secrete organic acids that erode tooth enamel. Pretty soon, a cavity appears which, under the constant exposure to these acids, gets deeper and deeper, finally invading the pulp of the tooth itself. So far, there are two elements involved in the production of dental caries: sugar and bacteria. A third element must also be considered—the hardness of the tooth enamel itself. Obviously the harder the enamel, the more resistant it will be to the acid secretions of the sugar-metabolizing bacteria. How hard a tooth becomes also depends to some extent on diet. Enamel, like bone, depends on calcium for its hardness. Unlike bone, however, enamel is not a reservoir except under extreme circumstances. Once formed, it holds on to its calcium. Thus, the crucial time for determining the hardness of the teeth is during early childhood when the teeth are forming.

Some studies have shown that a diet poor in calcium will result in poor enamel formation and in teeth that are extremely prone to cavities. It is important, therefore, that the diet of every young child be adequate in calcium. The time to begin is at birth. Breast milk is rich in calcium, which is in a form easily absorbed by the infant. If your infant is not being breast-fed, use a formula that is as close as possible to breast milk in composition. After the child is a year old, whole milk becomes the best source of calcium. If you are concerned about fat, low-fat or skim milk can replace whole milk at about eighteen months of age. Dairy products will continue to be the major source of dietary calcium throughout childhood, but as the child grows older, other foods can contribute significant amounts of it. See Table 23 in Chapter 8 for foods that are rich in calcium. Remember, taking in too much phosphorus will reduce calcium absorption. This is a particular problem in children, since many soft drinks contain significant amounts of phosphorus. Read the label; phosphoric acid means phosphorus. The child should substitute another drink without phosphoric acid.

Another very important nutrient in determining the hardness of teeth is fluoride, particularly during the early development of the teeth. Fluoride promotes calcium deposition, and ensures that it is firmly bound in the enamel. Fluoride is found in minute amounts in some foods and in some water supplies. In the United States many localities have added fluoride to their water supplies; others have not. There is no question that the addition of fluoride to water supplies has reduced the incidence of dental caries. However, many areas are still reluctant to fluoridate their water because of possible unknown side effects which theoretically could manifest themselves after long-term use. To date, we have not seen such effects. Fluoride is not present in breast milk in significant amounts, and therefore breast-fed babies should be supplemented with fluoride. Fluoride is not added to infant formula. Therefore, if you use powdered formulas and the water in your area is not fluoridated, your infant should be supplemented. Fluoride taken in small quantities into the body will get into the teeth only during the first year or so of life. However, when larger quantities are applied to the teeth they are effective throughout childhood. Therefore, the use of fluoridated toothpaste is recommended for all children.

To protect your youngster's teeth, then, the diet must be low in refined sugar, high in calcium, and relatively low in phosphorus, and during the first year of your child's life, have fluoride added to it either directly or through the water supply. But this type of diet is not enough because the form of the sugar in food may be even more important than the quantity of sugar consumed. If the sugar is supplied in a form that sticks to the teeth, such as chewing gum, caramels, candy bars, etc., it is much more dangerous than if it is in a form that quickly clears the mouth. Therefore, you must pay attention to how you consume your sugar, not just to how much you eat. If it is a sticky type, then it is a good idea to brush your teeth when you are finished.

The main points to remember in protecting yourself or your youngster from dental caries are:

- Brush frequently to reduce the bacterial count.
- Reduce the intake of refined sugar.
- Reduce the amount of sugar in a sticky form (and brush after you eat it).
- Take in an adequate supply of calcium.
- Reduce your phosphorus intake, particularly at the same time as you consume your calcium.
- Give your infant a fluoride supplement in the first year of life if you breast-feed or if the water supply in your area is not fluoridated.
- Brush with a fluoridated toothpaste.

Periodontal Disease

Periodontal disease is a condition that occurs in later life and doesn't really affect the teeth at all, but the gums and the bones into which the teeth are inserted. If left untreated, periodontal disease can lead first to a loosening of teeth and then to their loss. Periodontal disease is the major cause of tooth loss in older people, and it is the primary reason why such a high percentage of older people are toothless.

The cause or causes of periodontal disease are not clearly understood. Chronic infection of the gums is one part of the story. Erosion of the jawbones is another. Which comes first is not clear. Our best judgment is that in most cases the chronic infection leads to bone erosion. However, it is possible that in some cases the reverse is true. The erosion that occurs in the bones of the jaw is similar to that seen in osteoporosis. However, the risk factors associated with osteoporosis are not present in periodontal disease. It is not more frequent in women; it has no relation to menopause and it does not respond to hormone therapy. Thus, we cannot predict who will be at high risk for it.

Certainly good oral hygiene is very important in preventing periodontal disease. Frequent brushing, the use of mouthwashes, and dental flossing all contribute to the control of chronic infection of the gums. Frequent dental examinations will allow treatment to be started early if necessary so that the infection can be controlled before too much bone erosion has taken place.

Beyond this, however, there is a role for diet. As with the other bones of the body, the mandible and the maxilla (the two jawbones) participate in the regulation of body calcium. During early life, calcium is deposited in these bones; in later life, calcium loss occurs. The more calcium we can get into these bones, and the earlier, the more can be lost without seriously affecting bone structure later on. Thus, the same dietary principles that we discussed for osteoporosis are important in periodontal disease. Unlike osteoporosis, however, there is evidence that in some cases periodontal disease can actually be reversed by calcium supplementation. Although this approach does not work in many cases, it is worth trying, since there is little or no risk to taking a calcium supplement and the possible benefits may be great. The dosage should be between 500 and 1,000 mg daily in the form of calcium carbonate, calcium gluconate, or any nonphosphorus-containing calcium salt.

For Those at Low Risk

Suppose your risk for all the diseases we have discussed is low. Count your blessings! Even if this is true, however, there are reasons to consider changing your diet somewhat.

The fact that you are at low risk at any given time does not mean that you will remain at low risk for all time. Obviously, certain risk factors do not change—your sex, your race, your family history. Others, however, can change rapidly and sometimes dramatically. Suppose you have a serum cholesterol level of 160 and no other major risk factors for atherosclerosis. A year later you check your cholesterol level and it is 180; your risk is higher and the trend is in the wrong direction. Should you alter your diet and increase your activity? Certainly if your diet is high in fat and if your life-style is sedentary, the answer is yes. It is this changeability of risk factors in those diseases where risk can be clearly established, combined with our inability to define any specific risk factors in other diseases, that has prompted some experts to take what they consider a more global approach.

Recommendations from a number of prestigious sources have called for all Americans to change their diets. The argument given is that these changes will not harm us and may well benefit at least some of us. I cannot fully agree with that argument for several reasons. First, it discourages us from taking responsibility for a major part of our future health. Everyone should determine his or her own risk for those diseases in which such a determination is possible. If your risk is high, then certain changes in your diet may be indicated. If your risk is low, you must determine at regular intervals whether your risk has changed. This is your responsibility and no government nutrition guidelines are a substitute for discharging that responsibility.

Second, everyone does not have to change his or her diet even if risk factors cannot be established. Only those whose diet is poor in one respect or another need make certain changes. If you are a saltaholic, you should lower your salt intake; if your diet is high in fat, you should eliminate certain fatty foods. If you take in very little calcium or iron or zinc, you should take measures to correct the deficiency. While all these recommendations are appropriate for *many* people, they are not necessary for *all* people. Examine your own dietary pattern and then look at the recommendations. Make up your own mind as to what needs to be changed and how best to change it. The overall guidelines that have been recommended include:

Consuming the number of calories necessary to achieve and maintain ideal weight

Consuming no more than 30 percent of those calories in the form of fat

Taking in at least as much unsaturated fat as saturated fat

Keeping your salt (sodium) intake moderate

Consuming about 50 percent or slightly more of your calories as carbohydrate, with no more than 15 percent as simple sugar

Eating abundant quantities of foods containing dietary fiber

Look familiar? Some or all these guidelines have been designed for lowering your risk to one or a combination of diseases. Even if your risk is low they are worth considering if your present diet differs greatly. However, if you do decide to institute one or more of these changes, be careful not to unbalance your diet in such a way as to *increase* your risk for certain diseases. The woman who decides that she is taking in too much fat, particularly saturated fat, and cuts out all dairy products will lower her fat intake but may induce a calcium deficiency. Similarly, if she decides to cut out all meats, she may induce an iron deficiency. Radical changes in diet, particularly for those at low risk, should be avoided unless the diet is grossly abnormal, and if this is so, then those changes should be made in such a way as to ensure that the nutrient intake is balanced.

Finally, the first guideline in the list may not be appropriate for many people because in order to achieve and maintain ideal weight, they may have to struggle constantly with calories, thereby increasing their risk for other deficiencies. Perhaps a weight that is 105 percent of your ideal would be easier to achieve and maintain. As we have seen, it is just as healthy and may keep you from constantly dieting.

Clearly, in order for anyone to change his dietary pattern easily, adequate food choices must be available. While the United States has the most abundant food supply in the world, until recently our food choices with respect to nutrient content have been inadequate. Presently it is still not easy to lower your salt intake significantly. Of course, if you salt your food heavily you can stop. But what about the foods themselves? Until recently as their convenience went up, so did their salt content. TV dinners, canned foods, smoked or pickled foods were usually high in salt. Going on even a moderately salt-restricted diet meant a major change in life-style. It was difficult to eat in most restaurants or to take out food or snacks. Not so many years ago, this was true with respect to dietary fat. Today, however, there are many alternatives available: margarine, safflower or corn oil, skim milk, low-fat cheese. These foods did not appear by themselves, but because the public demanded them. The same is beginning to happen with low-salt foods, and if pressure kept up we will soon see a wide variety of high-fiber foods, whole-grain products, and foods rich in calcium, zinc, iron, and folic acid. Increasingly foods are being sold for the nutrients they contain—diet sodas for their low calories, salmon and sardines for their high-calcium content, chicken for its low-fat content, vegetables that are high in fiber, low-salt spaghetti sauce, and low-fat ice cream. Given the incentive of potentially large profits, the American food industry is extremely innovative—even low-salt potato chips are now available.

The more this trend continues, the easier it will become to alter your diet if you need to. Therefore, as more people participate in these dietary changes, the more choices become available, and those at high risk for certain diseases can make dietary changes more easily. At least, moving in the direction of the dietary guidelines outlined above will make it easier to alter your diet if necessary. Beyond that, as more and more products that conform to these guidelines become available, more and more people may find they like them. Our eating patterns may change totally. And who knows? Diet may no longer be a major risk factor for certain serious diseases.

Index